Doctor Kadans' Herbal Weight-Loss Diet

Also By the Author:

Encyclopedia of Fruits, Vegetables, Nuts and Seeds for Healthful Living, Parker Publishing Company Inc., 1973.

Modern Encyclopedia of Herbs, Parker Publishing Company, Inc., 1970.

Doctor Kadans' Herbal Weight-Loss Diet

DR. JOSEPH M. KADANS

Parker Publishing Company, Inc.
West Nyack, New York

© 1982 by

PARKER PUBLISHING COMPANY, INC.

West Nyack, N.Y.

This book is a reference work based on research by the author. The opinions
expressed herein are not necessarily those of or endorsed by the publisher. The
directions stated in this book are in no way to be considered as a substitute for
consultation with a duly licensed doctor.

Library of Congress Cataloging in Publication Data

Kadans, Joseph M.
   Doctor Kadans' herbal weight-loss diet.

   Includes index.
   1. Reducing diets.   2. Food, Natural.
3. Herbs.   I. Title.   II. Title: Herbal weight
loss diet.
RM222.2.K185   1982   613.2'5   82-7944
ISBN 0-13-216523-6   AACR2
ISBN 0-13-216531-7 (PBK)

PRINTED IN THE UNITED STATES OF AMERICA

Dedication

I wish to dedicate this book not only to my beloved wife, Adele, whose assistance and encouragement have been most helpful, but also to the large cadre of independent nutrition researchers, without axes to grind or products to sell, who have made exhaustive studies of food and food preparation and who have reduced their thoughts to writing. My own writing, speeches and work with people seeking to maintain good health or to regain it, have been greatly influenced by the writings of these devoted researchers, many of whom have been mentioned throughout this book. I would like to especially acknowledge the advice and wisdom of the late Lillian Buckin, my own dear mother-in-law, who lived a long and full life devoted to the studies of nature and natural living.

How This Book Will
Help You Lose Weight

I am proud to submit to readers interested in losing weight what I regard as the acme of excellence in a dieting program, one that is not only safe, but presents food intake as a series of constant adventures in interesting and delicious meals.

There are so many outstanding features in this book that it is impossible to list them all. For example, there is a section that tells you what foods you may feel free to nibble on during the day without any danger of gaining weight; another section tells the scientific truth about cholesterol, explaining why it is not as dangerous as many would have you believe it to be. Other parts of the book tell how diabetes can be avoided; how foods can be made delicious by the use of herbs and spices; an easy method for cleaning the colon; the secret of gaining energy without eating excessively; an explanation of sprout dieting; a description of harmful non-foods; which fats are needed and which should be avoided; an unusual "fun food"; and how to relax with herbs instead of coffee, tobacco or alcohol.

You will discover herb teas that are especially recommended for getting rid of excess fat. You will discover how you can avoid practically all illness by a special preparation of plant oil, prepared as a tea. You will learn how to mix the root of burdock with potatoes to get rid of fatty flesh. You'll read how another common root, available free in the fields and on the roadside, can be used as a healthy coffee substitute and at the same time rid the body of accumulations of fluid in body tissues.

In these pages you'll find out how to balance acid and alkaline foods so that your body fluids will not be too acid or too alkaline; you'll read how Helen H. returned to a normal weight and good health within 60 days; how Joan Y., 30, overweight and pregnant, got rid of constipation and excess pounds while at the same time giving her unborn baby the good nourishment needed for the right start in life; you'll learn about metabolism, the function of the thyroid and how to properly nourish that important gland.

To help you to get the daily intake of nutrients your body must have daily, you'll find a way of listing the nutrients you must have each day for a healthy and beautiful body. You will find ways of getting all of the needed vitamins and trace minerals at hardly any cost in Chapter 3.

You'll learn how Laura V., by merely changing her diet, slowed down the aging process and became a new person. You'll discover how to use a magic-like Oriental herb that for thousands of years has stood the test of time and proven itself again and again to be able to reverse the years. You'll discover a wonder herb that serves as a heart tonic, reduces high blood pressure as well as excess weight and helps the eyesight. This book tells you how to include these herbs in preparing your food.

You'll read how Kathy F. changed from a pudgy 165-pounder to a slim 120 pounds. Discover how Evelyn Y. used a common flavoring vegetable to regain her lost figure.

Do you think you need to count calories? You'll discover how Mary F. reduced her weight without counting calories.

You'll learn the secret of eating out, at the home of a friend or in a restaurant, without giving up your weight-losing diet. You'll discover how to determine what food supplements, vitamins or minerals you may need. You'll learn how to establish your own personal goal for weight loss. Discover for yourself the truth about roughage in the diet and the importance of thorough mastication.

You'll read how Robert B. rid himself of his huge paunch within two months. You'll read how Betty R. dropped from 185 pounds to 140 pounds within three months while eating delicious meals.

I describe how to steam your vegetables either in a steamer you can buy or in one that you can make yourself very easily. You'll learn how Evelyn T., a regular bread eater, used herbs in her bread and lost weight. I tell you how to prepare desserts that will not increase your weight and will still be delicious. And I include healthy and nonfat pies, cakes and cookies! Yes, and candy too, made of fruits, honey and nuts!

You'll discover how to use herbs in your bath water. This book tells you which herbs to use, how to use them and their effect upon your body. You'll also learn about the herb that is a sugar substitute and the herbs that will reduce your thirst for water, thereby preventing excessive drinking of fluids. You'll learn which herbs to use for inducing sound sleep.

Be sure to read what Sally C. has to say about broccoli. Sally tells how broccoli, with a few other foods, helps her to get her daily share of all the nutrients. The broccoli bonus for Sally was the help it gave her in reducing the size of her ankles.

I describe my own special vegetable cocktail that I prepare in a blender, helping me to maintain ideal weight and keeping me in excellent shape for tennis, and I explain the advantages and disadvantages of frozen and canned vegetables and fruits.

This book is the natural culmination of my efforts in first writing my herbal encyclopedia, *Modern Encyclopedia of Herbs,* and my fruit and vegetable book, *Encyclopedia of Fruits, Vegetables, Nuts and Seeds for Healthful Living,* both published by Parker Publishing Company. It has taken several years to prepare my new work but this final product combines the use of herbs, spices, fruits, vegetables, nuts and seeds into one treatise on careful food preparation so as to not only avoid the rocky shoals of excessive weight, so dangerous to health, but to guide the way to normal weight.

There are many other case histories and ideas in this book that make it a necessity for every home. It will be of great help to you and your family to attain good health and long life.

JOSEPH M. KADANS

Table of Contents

Doctor Kadans' Herbal Weight-Loss Diet

Chapter One

Modern
Health Researchers
Discover Herbs

And God said, "Behold, I have given you every herb-bearing seed that is upon the face of the earth."

Genesis 1:29

THE HERB is truly a God-given gift, considering its many valuable uses for healing the body and its use as a flavoring for food improvement.

It is perhaps strange to note that billions of dollars have been spent and are still being spent to help researchers find highly technical and complex cures for diseases and for prevention of illness by immunization. Yet we are slowly but surely coming to the conclusion that simple herbs and spices, used constantly even before Biblical days, not only cure and prevent disease but lend a tang and taste to food that makes every meal an adventure and every day a joy.

Strange as it may seem, you will find that many herbs contain nutritional elements needed by your body, thus making it important to include herbs in your diet. Herbs have healing qualities and are safe to use. For example, natural licorice has been reported as useful for healing ulcers in the duodenum.

Delicious herbal teas, you'll discover, are an excellent substitute for coffee and regular teas, which contain caffeine, a dangerous drug. Herb teas can be prepared from either fresh or dry herb leaves, roots, seeds or flowers. A teaspoon of the dried herb is usually enough for a cup. It is best, of course, to first steep the tea in a tea pot, pour boiling water over the herb and allow it to steep for about ten minutes. You should use a strainer to then pour the tea into a teacup and, if desired, add honey and lemon for taste. For a summer drink, allow it to cool in the refrigerator or add ice cubes. These drinks are much healthier than the soft drinks containing caffeine or the hard drinks containing alcohol. (Beer is also alcoholic and should be avoided.)

This book is not intended to be a medical home-remedy book and does not dwell on the medicinal values of herbs, but I cannot avoid telling you that you will benefit greatly from the use of herbs in your diet. At the same time you will be able to restrict your food intake to healthy foods which, with the addition of herbs and spices in your diet, will not only greatly lengthen your life span but will add tasty and spicy foods that will make eating a delight.

HOW AN EFFICIENT DIET
REQUIRES LESS FOOD INTAKE

The wonderful part of a well-guided diet program is that less food is required to satisfy your appetite. As a result, you will experience two distinct benefits. First, the organs and glands of your body will need to do less work and second, the cost of your food will be less.

The stomach is an amazing chemical laboratory. Adding various food substances into the stomach produces various chemical changes. Each morsel of food, depending upon whether it is acid or alkaline, solid or liquid, sweet or sour, fresh or stale or whether it is any of a large number of various identifiable substances, reacts differently in the stomach. When you eat only pure, simple and fresh foods, you keep the work of your body chemical laboratory to a minimum.

An overweight person often has an overdistended, flabby stomach. If you reduce the amount of food you eat, your stomach gradually contracts to its normal size and your flabby stomach becomes a relic of the past. One result of a normal-sized stomach is that there soon disappears the hunger rumblings that result in a fast walk to the refrigerator to avoid what seems to be an early demise due to starvation.

Just as a good homemaker establishes a budget and does not exceed it, allotting a proportion of the income for food, another portion for clothing and another portion for shelter, etc., so does the good dieter arrange for foods that will meet the daily needs of the body for vitamins, minerals, proteins, carbohydrates and fats.

As an efficient dieter, you will make certain that you care for all of the needs of your body daily, and that these needs are in your daily "budget," but you will not "overspend" so as to take in more of the nutritional elements than you need.

The dieter who spends beyond his or her budget and stuffs the body with unneeded food is clearly wasting valuable food resources and over-working the body organs and glands. Even assuming that the dieter has unlimited finances to purchase unlimited quantities and varieties of foods, it is nevertheless unwise to burden the body with unnecessary work.

If you want to obtain the maximum use of your bodily functions, you will have to change your old habits of eating whenever and whatever your fancy desires.

NIBBLING AT WILL VS. REGULAR MEALS

Experienced people in the field of nutrition know that nibbling at will can be dangerous. However, this is only true when the articles nibbled are fattening, contain injurious substances or constitute a burden on an already overloaded body.

Nibbling on a piece of celery, for example, may not be bad at all. It may satisfy your craving for food during a time in early dieting when your mind is not yet adjusted to a program of eating and drinking only what is good and necessary. To have to wait for the regular mealtime may be too much of a strain for the beginning dieter.

Another good item for nibbling is an apple or an orange. By all means, avoid donuts, cakes, pizza, hamburgers, coffee, soft drinks, ice cream, candy or the like. This kind of nibbling is definitely dangerous.

A snack of carrots, either raw or in the form of juice, is an excellent item for nibbling and will do wonders for the skin and for the eyesight because of its high vitamin A content. If you should see someone with a ruddy glow on the cheeks, the chances are that he or she eats lots of carrots or drinks carrot juice.

Another good item for occasional nibbling is sunflower seeds. If you have been accustomed to a coffee break or a cola break, you will find that taking a few sunflower seeds will break you of the coffee or cola habit. Sunflower seeds are usually about 25 percent protein and this protein "lift" can well replace the lifted feeling you get from coffee or tea, which contain caffeine and therefore should be avoided.

There is no need to forego the regular three meals a day, with or without between-meal nibbling. The ideal, of course, is to include all the required nutrients within the three meals. Careful planning of meals is necessary in order to include all the necessary nutrients and in proper quantity—not too little and not too much.

By the time you finish reading this book, you should learn what to include and what to omit from your food and drink.

WHAT SARAH C. LEARNED ABOUT CHOLESTEROL

Sarah C., 38, had read so many frightening things about the dangers of cholesterol that she decided that she would scrupulously avoid all foods containing it. Little did she realize that it was like trying to run from her own shadow.

The old adage about a little knowledge being dangerous is as true as it ever was. I explained to Sarah that the body actually makes more than five times as much cholesterol as the amount one is likely to eat. It is the eating of sugar that is the culprit and not the foods that are rich in cholesterol such as liver, brains and egg yolk. Most people eat too much sugar and products made with sugar. I explained to Sarah that the body makes cholesterol from fatty acids, but also makes cholesterol from amino acids and sugar products. Amino acids are protein elements and, as there is some protein in most all foods, the body can make as much cholesterol as it wants.

I also informed Sarah that the organ foods such as liver and brains are excellent nutritional sources. So are eggs. Instead of eliminating these foods from her diet, she was told to eliminate all sugar from her diet, including hidden sugar sources such as honey, molasses and fruits. Also, she was told to limit severely her intake of carbohydrates such as bread or potatoes. Finally, she was asked to exercise daily, even if it was only a walk around the block.

Before beginning her diet, Sarah weighed 138 pounds and was five feet two inches tall. According to standard height and weight tables, her weight should have been about 130 pounds; consequently, she was only slightly overweight.

Her problem, therefore, was not her weight but rather her condition. She was easily fatigued, somewhat nervous and irritable, had frequent headaches, caught colds occasionally and was constipated usually just prior to her monthly periods.

I told Sarah not to worry about cholesterol; a low cholesterol diet deprived her of many good foods rated very high in vitamins and minerals, such as egg yolks. This alone relieved much of her anxiety and reduced considerably her nervousness and irritability. The reduction in tension and a well-rounded diet program eliminated her headaches, colds and constipation. Within a month, she was a different woman. Results were noticeable even after a week.

Sarah started eating two eggs daily with a breakfast of two slices of whole wheat toast, some oatmeal with low-fat milk and a glass of freshly-made orange juice. The eggs were boiled for four minutes after the water started boiling.

For lunch, she would have either a lettuce and tomato sandwich on rye or whole wheat toast, or would make a sandwich out of Swiss or muenster cheese with some lettuce. A tuna fish sandwich was also a favorite with her.

There are of course an infinite variety of food combinations that would be satisfactory for a light and satisfying lunch. For example, instead of a sandwich, a milk-vegetable soup can be easily prepared. For one serving, slice an onion and chop two or three slices, depending upon the size of the onion. Chop a stalk of celery and one small carrot. Cook until tender in one cup of low-fat or skimmed milk. Add some herbal spices such as paprika, chives or parsley.

Sarah was not a vegetarian, so I advised her to prepare her fish and meat dinners by either broiling or roasting. When broiling, she was told to use a broiler with a rack so that the meat or fish would not soak up the fat that dropped from the food.

When eating potatoes with her meals, Sarah was advised to limit the butter and sour cream to a minimum and to either boil or bake the potatoes. She was told to refrain from any frying of potatoes and to especially avoid the so-called french-fried variety.

She often ate fish, preparing it by "poaching" the fish in the manner that eggs are poached. Sarah simply brought water to a boil and then placed the fish in the water and let it cook for a few minutes, enough to tenderize it. The herb known as asafetida is generally recognized as a favorite for flavoring of fish, meats and soups. Also, cloves are excellent for sprinkling over fish, eggs, potatoes and tomatoes.

The diet program for Sarah could well be adopted by many others, with or without her symptoms. As for drinking with meals, Sarah was told to avoid coffee and the ordinary teas and to drink herb teas, made with such herbs and spices as clover flowers, alfalfa, peppermint, roasted chicory, catnip or chamomile flowers.

The ideal diet is to avoid canned or processed foods and to have sufficient variety so as to include all of the necessary vitamins, minerals, carbohydrates and fats in sufficient amounts to meet the needs of the body.

HOW HERBS AND SPICES HELPED MINERVA E. WITH HER DIET

Minerva E. consulted me at the age of 27. She was considerably overweight, since she was only five feet six inches tall and weighed 185 pounds. She had tried dieting many times, but she claimed all her diets were so tasteless and dull that she could not continue them. She would lose weight whenever she dieted, but after some weight loss Minerva would return to her former eating habits and gain it all back again.

After I listened to her sad story of repeated failures, I convinced her that dieting was not enough—she must change her whole way of living. Minera would have to stay away from unhealthy foods for good, and eat nutritious meals, overcoming her lack of interest in diet foods by adding herbs and spices to all of her meals.

Minerva's biggest problem was her strong desire for pies, rolls, cakes, breads and other baked goods. Cookies were her special delight. I explained to her that bakery products are heavily loaded with carbohydrates, and that cakes, cookies and pies are excessively rich in sugar. I warned Minerva that if she continued eating foods full of carbohydrates and sugars it would lead her to an early grave.

She believed me and changed her meals at once. This was the turning point in her life. In less than two weeks, Minerva experienced a substantial weight loss. She stuck to her diet and continued to lose weight gradually but steadily, week after week, until within six months she had reduced to 135 pounds.

As part of her education in eating, I told Minerva how an excessive intake of carbohydrates such as sugar made her pancreas produce excessive insulin. Her intake of large amounts of sugar would wear out her pancreas so it could not manufacture. Then, when a shortage of insulin occurred, the glucose remained in the blood stream.

Insulin would ordinarily convert the glucose to glycogen, which would be stored in the liver. By the lack of insulin, with the glucose remaining in the blood stream, the kidneys would pass the glucose into the urine. In addition, the heavy loading of the blood stream with glucose would cause tissues throughout the body, reached by the tiny blood vessels known as capillaries, to become flooded with glucose and then fail to function normally.

Minerva became convinced of the importance of avoiding excessive carbohydrates. The next step was to make her new diet program so interesting that she would not want to leave it even after she achieved her weight loss.

The use of herbs and spices was the answer. For breakfast, I suggested that Minerva sprinkle ground cloves and paprika over her eggs and lightly buttered whole wheat toast. She tried it and loved it.

For lunch, I encouraged Minerva to have some yogurt with fresh fruit such as cantaloupe, peaches or bananas. Papaya is also an excellent fruit. The mixture is then sprinkled with nutmeg before serving to give it a novel and exciting taste.

I told Minerva to confine herself to moderate amounts of meat and potatoes and when she ate potatoes to eliminate bread from the menu. She was told about the use of ginger to sprinkle over broiled or baked fish, pot roast, steak, lamb, veal, carrots or onions. Ginger imparts a spicy flavor to foods and has the wonderful side effect of preventing colds and stomach gases.

Minerva had a strong urging for soft drinks, especially cola drinks. When I explained to her about the caffeine in cola drinks as well as in soft drinks generally, she agreed to stop using soft drinks and to start using herb teas made from such herbs as ginseng, peppermint, catnip or chamomile. For hot weather, I told her how the tea, after sweetening with some honey and lemon juice for flavoring, could be cooled and made into a tasty drink.

By removing the high carbohydrate diet from her regimen, Minerva started losing weight slowly but regularly. She reached her ideal weight goal after six months, losing about two pounds per week regularly.

Incidentally, I also urged Minerva to do more walking as a form of exercise. This was of great help in getting rid of excess poundage.

CLEANING OUT THE SYSTEM BEFORE DIETING

In cases of substantial overweight, I advise people in lectures and in personal consultations to clean out their lower bowels with enemas or colonics. Unfortunately, within the bodies of many people, a poor diet over many years has resulted in the formation of encrustations over the internal lining of the small and large intestines.

There are normally tiny hairy projections in the lining of the digestive tract, which act to propel the contents of the intestines toward the final outlet. The crustaceous coating interferes with the utilization of these tiny hairy projections.

It does little good to eat fresh and nourishing foods when, after leaving the stomach itself, where the digestion starts, the remainder of the journey of these foods through the digestive system is largely wasted. The value of the foods is limited because of the encrustations that have formed over the years, which prevent the nutrients from being absorbed by the capillaries and into the blood circulation system.

It is hard for many people to realize that they might have a partial occlusion or blocking of the digestive tract, because they know that they have regular bowel movements. However, post-mortem studies have revealed that these partial intestinal blockages exist in many individuals, similar to the partial blocking of blood vessels in the condition known as arteriosclerosis or hardening of the arteries.

We have not yet found a way to wash out the hardened arteries, but we have long ago learned that the intestinal tract, especially the lower bowels, can be fairly well cleaned out by enemas or colonic irrigations. This is not usually accomplished with one flushing but may take a series of cleanings. In most every large city there are professional men and women who specialize in giving enemas or colonics to clean out the lower bowels.

Perhaps an important reason why so many people are overweight and obese is because of inadequate function of the absorbent processes of the digestive system. Much food they eat ought to be ingested, but instead passes through the digestive system largely undigested. This leaves the body cells undernourished and consequently there is that feeling of hunger that causes the individual to keep eating until that hungry feeling is satisfied, even if this means overeating.

It is plain that for a diet program to be truly effective, the digestive system must be in sound condition. Just as water pipes often acquire a buildup of rust and sediment, thus narrowing the amount of water that actually passes through, so does the opening of the intestines gradually narrow so that while evacuations may continue, the amount of the evacuation is limited by the small size of the intestinal passage.

Also, it is generally recognized that the substance comprising the buildup may also consist of undigested food particles which, when originally swallowed, may have been fit for digestion but over the passage of time were transformed into an inedible toxic substance. This substance, in contact with the very thin capillary system of blood vessels, is being constantly absorbed into the blood stream and body tissues throughout the body, spreading poisons into all body parts, joints, organs and glands.

It is therefore of prime importance, at the start of any diet program, to first clean out the digestive tract and to especially remove clogging and impurities from the lower bowels. Only after a cleaning out will the body mechanism be able to function properly.

HOW ELEANOR T. CONTROLLED
HER URGE TO SNACK

Eleanor T. had just reached her 55th birthday when she paid me a visit to consult about her overweight. She was five feet, five inches tall and weighed 185 pounds, about 25 percent over the average for a person of her age and height.

I planned a program of meals for her similar to the program outlined for Sarah C., previously mentioned in this chapter. After two or three follow-up visits, although there was some weight control improvement noticed, it was not good enough. After some close questioning, I discovered her trouble. Eleanor had a problem she could not control. She would develop a strong hunger for food between meals and it seemed like nothing could keep her away from that refrigerator, looking for snacks.

She would look for and devour anything in the refrigerator resembling food. She claimed that she had followed my instructions in every way except for snacking between meals. Of course, snacking away as she did, without regard to calories, almost nullified all of her other good eating regimen. Later in this chapter, I will discuss selective snacking and how to snack without danger. As for Eleanor, we solved her snacking problem completely so that she did not do any snacking at all.

The first step was to increase the amount of protein in Eleanor's diet, so that she would have plenty of energy to continue with her day's activities without tiring. She was told to have one-half grapefruit for breakfast, then two eggs and some hot cereal such as oatmeal or some whole wheat cereal, and two slices of toasted whole wheat bread. To add to her nourishment for the morning, she could also drink a cup of whole milk.

With such a full breakfast, she had no need for an in-between snack. Eleanor was especially prone to chocolate candy bars for snacking and this is usually an indication of the need for additional protein in the diet.

For lunch, I told Eleanor she could partake of a large serving portion of meat, fish or fowl. Also, she could have a choice of three vegetables such as a baked potato, string beans, peas, lettuce, tomato, corn, rice or any one of a number of other nourishing foods. Green lettuce should always be included in both the lunch and dinner meals and possibly celery, green peppers and onions, if available and in season.

Eleanor was also urged to remove some pounds by taking a walk daily or swimming or playing tennis. An hour's walk will burn away 200 calories while an hour of tennis will consume about 400 calories. A half hour of swimming uses an additional 200 calories.

I explained the calorie system to Eleanor. Food represents energy and energy represents calories. We need calories for our daily activities and by activities we also mean brain activities such as studying or conversing. If we use up more calories than what we ingest in our foods, we lose weight because the body then obtains the calories needed from reserve stores of fat and protein.

To make certain that her hunger was fully satisfied after the luncheon and dinner meals, Eleanor was urged to make a large vegetable salad for each of these meals. She was told to cut up half a green pepper and combine it with one-third of a cup of chopped carrots. To this could be added a cup of chopped cabbage, a few chunks of zucchini, some thin slices of turnip, some lettuce and a few slices of tomatoes.

With three full meals and plenty of low calorie vegetables to eat, Eleanor lost her urge to snack between meals. Her weight went down and her feeling of well-being went up.

DAVID R.'S EXPERIENCE WITH A MACROBIOTIC DIET

David R. had a friend who had gone on a macrobiotic diet. In a consultation about David's obesity, David told me that he wanted to try a macrobiotic diet also.

Macro means large, while micro refers to very small elements. The word "biotic" refers to life. Therefore, a macrobiotic diet refers to a diet that has a very large amount of live foods.

David was 44 years old and weighed 275 pounds at the time I got him started on this macrobiotic diet. He was only five feet eight inches tall and according to the weight tables his proper weight should have been not more than 190 pounds.

My first step was to have David take a series of colonic cleanings. There was no reason why he could not start on his macrobiotic diet at the same time he was taking these treatments.

Which are the foods with life? There are no foods livelier than sprouts! I devised a regimen of foods which included sprouted foods for David, and it worked beautifully. He experienced improvement in less than a week. Adding some sprouts to his meals, David lost two pounds the first week, three pounds the next and for the next nine months lost two or three pounds a week until his weight was down to normal for his age and height, 190 pounds.

Sprouts can supply your body's nutritional needs in ample quantities and in easily assimilable form. Best of all, they are easily available at extremely low cost throughout the year. You do not need a garden to grow your own sprouts. While there are many sprouting devices, the most simple is to take a jar and soak some seeds suitable for sprouting overnight. In the morning, pour out the water and leave the moist seeds to sprout, laying the jar on its side to make more space for the sprouts to grow. In the late afternoon, rinse the sprouts with water, pour out the water and allow the seeds to sprout a little more. Repeat the process twice a day, morning and late afternoon, until the sprouts are ready to be eaten.

I explained the sprouting method to David and he agreed to it, but instead of late afternoon he did the rinsing in the early evening, which was all right. He decided to try alfalfa seed, mung beans and sunflower seeds. To make sure that the seeds or dried beans would be fresh and unsprayed, I advised David to buy them from a health food store. Other seeds suitable for sprouting are soybeans, fenugreek, peas, wheat and sesame seeds.

To insure having sufficient sprouts every day, David was told to start a new bath of sprouts every day for a week. Then, as each batch was eaten daily, there would be a new batch ready for the next day's use.

I instructed David to use sprouts with every meal. For example, sprouts can be added to soft boiled eggs just before serving, to make a live breakfast with live enzymes. For use with scrambled eggs, sprouts could be added to the pan after the eggs are ready and the fire is turned off. Be careful not to heat the sprouts to the extent that the live enzymes would be destroyed, which usually occurs at a temperature of 140° F.

For lunch and dinner, David was told to use the sprouts in many ways. For example, they could be added to soups, stews, souffles or placed in a blender with other vegetables to make a healthy vegetable drink. While the ideal way is to eat them raw or warmed but not excessively heated, sprouts may be cooked with meat loaves or in casseroles and still provide many minerals and vitamins even after the heat destroys the live enzymes.

David was also told how to make fresh fruit and vegetable juices. He was fortunate enough to have a little garden space, so I urged David to purchase a few comfrey roots and to grow them in his garden. The young leaves are delicious when eaten raw and may also be used in vegetable drinks with other plants such as parsley, mint or alfalfa. Papaya ranks high in enzymes and is a delicious fruit.

With the combination of the usual diet for dieters intent on reducing and this type of macrobiotic diet, with large amounts of live foods, David used the live sprouts, many of them of herbal nature, together with live fruit and vegetable drinks, to find his way to good health, long life and happiness.

ARNOLD P.'S WAY OF LOWERING HIS PROTEIN INTAKE

Arnold P. was tall and muscular and weighed 230 pounds. He was five feet nine inches tall and at age 37 he could be considered to be about 35 pounds overweight.

When I questioned Arnold about his eating habits, I found that he was eating far too much protein but that most of his other eating and drinking habits were not far off balance. We therefore concentrated on reducing his protein intake.

The general rule about protein intake is to eat an amount equivalent to about one gram daily for every two pounds of weight. For an individual weighing 230 pounds, therefore, the protein intake should be 115 grams per day. As the weight decreased, so should the intake of protein.

In checking into Arnold's eating habits, I found that he enjoyed eating ham and eggs, bacon and eggs or a small steak and eggs for breakfast. A serving of bacon (two slices) is equal to about 35 grams; a ham or steak serving would be about 20 grams.

Eggs have about 12 grams of protein each. Since Arnold ate three eggs with his breakfast, this would amount to 36 grams. Two slices of whole wheat toast would amount to an additional 24 grams, at 12 grams for each slice.

The orange juice he drank each morning had 1 or less than a gram of protein, so he could disregard the protein content of the orange juice.

A breakfast of bacon and eggs, therefore, would amount to 35 plus 36 plus 24, for a total of 95 grams. This was only for breakfast, yet already he was close to the maximum of 115 grams for the day. Let us see what he consumed in protein for lunch and for dinner.

Arnold always had a vegetable salad for lunch, which usually included some lettuce, celery, parsley, carrots and cucumber slices. This would be sometimes topped with yogurt. As lunches go, this is close to the ideal lunch for anyone.

Except for the parsley, which rates at 3 grams for a serving, the other vegetables rated only as 1 gram each, for a total of 7 grams.

Arnold would have done well with a 7-gram protein lunch but he would usually include some fried chicken with his lunch or a hamburger, which would add an additional 25 grams of protein to the lunch for a total protein lunch of 32 grams.

These 32 grams added to the 95 grams for breakfast came to a total of 127 grams; Arnold had already exceeded the total number of 115 grams allowable for the day without even counting his evening meal! And oh yes, we must add about 8 grams for the roll that he would eat with his hamburger or chicken, bringing the total to 135 grams.

For dinner, Arnold would often eat a steak or a leg of lamb, which would account for an additional 75 grams of protein or thereabouts. A baked potato would amount to only about 2 grams; some tomatoes and peas would amount to 1 gram and 3 grams of protein respectively.

If he ate some fish for dinner instead of meat, his protein intake would be about 20 grams instead of 75. Arnold did eat fish occasionally but he preferred meat.

Arnold would also eat two or three slices of bread and butter with his dinner. Although the protein content of butter is negligible (less than 1 gram per serving), the bread averaged 10 or 12 grams of protein each slice, depending upon the kind of bread. Arnold preferred whole wheat and so at 12 grams per slice, this added 24 to 36 grams to his dinner. Most of the time, he would be content with two slices, so let us add 24 grams to the total.

From what we have counted thus far, the total number of grams of protein Arnold would ordinarily consume for dinner would be 105 grams.

Arnold also loved cream of mushroom soup, which unfortunately for him, is rich in protein, with about 36 grams to a serving. This would make the total 141 grams for dinner.

With 127 grams of protein for breakfast and lunch and about 141 grams for dinner, this gave Arnold a total of 268 grams of protein for the day or an excess of 153 grams of protein.

Arnold admitted that occasionally he got out of bed and raided the icebox for a snack, such as a cold chicken leg (28 grams) or a glass of milk (15 grams). On the days he indulged in these delights he increased his protein intake that much more.

I advised Arnold to make a number of changes in his meals. Arnold was told to eliminate one egg from his breakfast and one slice of toast; also, to eliminate all meat from breakfast. His breakfast reduction would amount to 59 grams.

At lunch, Arnold continued eating salads and yogurt but eliminated his fried chicken or hamburger with roll, so he saved 33 grams of protein.

For dinner, Arnold ate fish instead of meat and saved an additional 35 grams of protein. By eliminating the two slices of bread and butter, he saved an extra 24 grams of protein. By eliminating the cream of mushroom soup he prevented the absorption of an additional 36 grams of protein into his digestive system.

By eliminating these foods, Arnold saved a total of 163 grams of protein. Since his original consumption was 153 grams in excess, the elimination of 163 grams would be more than enough to bring him down to normal.

During a diet, foods must be carefully selected so that they will contain all of the necessary vitamins and minerals as well as protein, carbohydrates and fats needed by the body. Arnold was duly warned to make certain that he had enough of a variety in his food intake so that all of the nutrients needed by his body would be provided.

By eliminating all snacks and the unnecessary protein foods from his diet, Arnold felt better within two weeks and started to show improvement in his weight less than a week after his dieting started.

He was encouraged to eat soups low in protein content such as tomato, green pea, cream of celery or cream of asparagus.

Arnold was also taught how to make hot and cold beverages from herb teas such as spearmint, chamomile, alfalfa and clover flowers. To add taste to his salads, he was told to sprinkle them with one or more of herbs such as anise, catnip, chervil, chives, cumin seeds, garlic, hyssop, mace, tarragon vinegar and thyme.

He was encouraged to sprinkle his fish dishes with asafetida, basil, chervil, cloves, ginger, mace, marjoram, nutmeg, oregano, rosemary and turmeric

To lend a delightful flaver to his meat selections, I advised him to use one or more of these herbs: asafetida, basil, bay leaves, cinnamon, cloves, cumin seeds, garlic, ginger, mace, marjoram, nutmeg, paprika, tarragon vinegar, thyme and turmeric.

To vent his appetite for snacks, he was encouraged to maintain a supply of apples. It would take five apples to equal one gram of protein. Apples are indeed a low protein food.

In less than six months after starting his new diet program, Arnold had reduced to a normal weight of 145 pounds and he was feeling more fit than ever before in his life.

ELIMINATING NON-FOODS FROM THE DIET

First, what is meant by non-foods and second, why eliminate them from the diet?

Non-foods means things that we swallow, whether solid or liquid, that have no nutritional value. Some argument could be made that even ordinary water has nutritional value and is not, therefore, a "non-food." The nutritional value would consist, according to this argument, in liquefying what would otherwise be a dry food and difficult, if not impossible, to digest.

Scientific studies by nutritionists have shown that, despite popular belief to the contrary, it is not necessary to have drinks accompany solid foods if the proper foods are eaten. Most natural foods consist of water and the water in the food, plus the salivary juices, is generally sufficient liquid for ideal digestion and assimilation.

The right kind of food is alive and gives live energy to the body. When food has been processed to the point where important minerals and vitamins have either been destroyed or removed, such a food becomes a non-food. Sweet rolls, donuts, dumplings, candy, cola drinks and, generally speaking, foods that have been fried, stewed, boiled or preserved may all be considered as non-foods. The more the food is processed the more it is converted from a live food to a non-food.

Everyone should try to go on a program of nutrition wherein naturally prepared foods will be the mainstay of the diet and non-foods kept to a minimum.

THE NEED FOR SOME FAT IN THE DIET

Some people might think all fats are non-foods. The body does need fat, however. A layer of fat serves as a cushion for protection from bumps and bruises, helps keep the body warm and can be helpful to the skin. If care is taken to ingest only the unsaturated fatty acids from vegetable oils, the skin is apt to be clear and healthy.

There is danger, of course, in excessive fat. Besides the extra burden on the heart in having to work harder to carry the extra weight, excessive fat in the diet inhibits the secretion of the gastric juice and thereby delays the digestion of food.

There are some fat formations found naturally in such foods as meat, fish, avocados, nuts, egg yolks, sunflower seeds and many other foods but such fats are usually easily digestible and safe, if not taken to excess degrees.

What we need to avoid are the fats found in fried foods, heavy salad dressings, rich pastries, butter, cheese and some fish. Bacon and other pork foods are generally extremely rich in fat content and should be indulged in rarely if at all.

A small amount of fat is needed by the body to meet the need for energy. Fat reserves are used for energy when there is a scarcity of dextrose or sweets.

A little fat is fine but an excessive amount is bad!

MERRILY, WE SNACK ALONG

Snacking? Am I kidding? No! Snacking is OK if it is the right kind. Also, an important benefit is that it will keep hunger pangs away so that when you sit down for a meal you will limit your portions to what is actually needed and not eat merely for the pleasure of eating.

Just what is the right kind of snack? One of the ideal snacking treats is nibbling on a raw carrot. No nutrition expert will say this is bad for you any time or any place!

A raw carrot is richly endowed with vitamin A and also has some of the B vitamins as well as vitamin C. It has value as food energy and has protein, carbohydrates and some fat. The carrot is also amply supplied with minerals such as calcium, phosphorus, iron, sodium and potassium. Keep a carrot or two in a little plastic bag in your pocket or purse and encourage members of your family to do the same.

Snacking on apples is a good habit, too. Although not as heavily loaded with vitamin C as the carrot, the apple has about the same quantity of other vitamins, minerals, protein, carbohydrate and fat as the carrot.

Eating an orange for a snack also gives you a natural lift that is far superior to a cola drink or coffee.

What's wrong with coffee for a snack? Coffee does have some food energy value and also has some minerals such as calcium, phosphorus, iron, sodium and potassium. It also has a small amount of riboflavin and niacin, part of the B complex vitamins. However, coffee is a harsh drink because of the caffeine content and, generally speaking, is harmful to the kidneys and to the heart. The caffeine is a bitter crystalline alkaloid generally used as a stimulant and as a diuretic. Caffeine is also found in tea, except in herbal teas.

Never snack on a sweet roll! The sugar in the sweet roll or covering it in the form of an icing or as a jelly is the culprit. Sugar is a deceitful enemy. Pretending to be your friend by making you happy with the sweet taste, sugar robs your bones and tissues of vital elements, taking away important nutrients as it travels throughout the body in the blood stream. Using sugar results in a form of cannibalism where your own body is devoured by itself and excreted through the kidneys and the urine.

Sure! Go ahead and snack between meals, but make sure that it is something helpful and not harmful.

TOM B.'S METHOD OF CLEANING OUT HIS SYSTEM

No matter what diet he tried, Tom B. could not lose weight. He tried every conceivable eating program but nothing seemed to work. Tom weighed 260 pounds and was only five feet, six inches tall. When I met him, Tom had just reached his 35th birthday.

A study of his diet revealed Tom was ingesting an excessive amount of white bread, meat, potatoes, spaghetti, meat balls, fried foods, coffee and beer. While the potatoes themselves would not be bad, as potatoes are not dangerous, he always loaded them heavily with butter. Half the time, he ate them in the form of french-fried potatoes, a serving containing 274 calories, as compared with a baked potato, which contains only 93 calories.

Following my theory that overweight people often need to eat because they are not properly assimilating the food they swallow, I recommended that Tom B. take a colonic as a cleansing of his large bowel or intestine. This is best done with colonics although there are herbs that do a fairly good cleansing. One of the most commonly used herbs is cascara sagrada.

There are also certain vegetables that cleanse as well as nourish. Some vegetables recommended for their cleansing effect are carrots, celery, collard greens, corn, peas, potatoes, radishes, rhubarb, summer squash, tomatoes and turnips.

For the first two weeks of his new regimen, Tom took at least one colonic each day and concentrated on eating the vegetables I recommended to him. I did not allow Tom to eat without restraint although it is commonly believed that superior foods may be eaten without limit. This is a fallacy. Only enough food should be consumed to satisfy the needs of the body. Anything more is gluttony.

It took only three days for Tom to start losing weight and thereafter he lost almost a pound a day for the next three weeks. He gradually started to return to a more normal diet but avoided all canned and processed foods and foods containing sugar, coffee, tea, cola drinks, candy, ice cream, cakes, cookies, pies and donuts.

Tom agreed with me that it was very likely his large intestines or bowels were overly obstructed with dried colonic contents. This had at least two undesirable effects. First, it created an interference with meals being absorbed through the walls of the intestines. Second, the fecal matter, not passing through the intestines, developed a toxicity which transmitted toxic materials into the blood stream. Of course, the blood travels throughout the body into all tissues, glands and organs, carrying either nutritive elements such as oxygen, protein, vitamins and minerals, or dangerous substances of a toxic nature that may be dangerous enough to overcome the body's natural resistance to disease.

The lesson Tom learned can be applied to many cases of excessive weight, where ordinary diets do not seem to help.

GRADUAL CHANGES IN EATING HABITS ARE BEST

There is no need for you to be uncomfortable at the start of your new diet program. Gradual changes are best.

Once you decide to go on a diet, make plans for some minor deviations now and then. For instance, although butter is very fattening, you may not want to eliminate it entirely from the diet at the very start. Allow yourself a little butter on your toast in the morning but spread it very thin. Then, avoid butter the rest of the day. This rule also applies to margarine. While there are many who consider margarine to be a good substitute for butter, it just isn't so. Official government food tables show that there are 716 calories in an edible portion of butter and that there are 720 calories in an equal amount of margarine. So, for someone who wishes to cut down on calories, the substitution of margarine for butter is not the answer.

Recently, yogurt has become popular as a substitute for ice cream. This is a good diet variation to make your dieting easier. Yogurt can be easily made with skimmed milk or with low-fat powdered milk. Perhaps the easiest way is to bring the milk almost to a boil and then let it cool to a point where it is warm and yet not cold. Pour the milk into small containers and place them in the oven at the lowest oven temperature—enough to keep them warm. It will take about three or four hours for the yogurt to jell into a semi-solid form. One important factor must not be overlooked. You must stir into your milk during the heating period about two or three tablespoons of "starter" yogurt, to help your new yogurt get started.

In adopting yogurt as a fun-food substitute for fatty ice cream, beware of the sugar-rich flavoring that is used in yogurt flavors on the market. Make your yogurt plain and if you buy yogurt, get the plain and avoid the kind with flavoring.

One of the best ways to change easily into a diet program is to gradually reduce the quantity of the food you eat. This has a double purpose. First, it tends to reduce the size of your stomach. When your stomach shrinks a little, it reduces your appetite because the stomach fills up more quickly, giving you that satisfied feeling earlier. Second, you avoid overworking the body organs when you do not overload the body's digestive machinery. This allows the organs to maintain good health. Constant overworking of organs wears out the body and is a contributing factor in many cases of early demise.

BECOMING SLIM WITH THE HELP OF NATURE

Is it not the purpose of proper food intake, known as dieting, to stay healthy or to improve your health? Of course! That is why it is so important for you to partake of the best foods available. Avoid foods that have been largely devitalized as the result of *processing,* the term used to disguise the practice of treating foods by removing ingredients that spoil easily and thereby prevent a long life on the grocery shelves. Important vitamins needed by the body are removed so that the final product will look better and last longer on the shelves.

Some of the foods that have been "watered down" are flour, sugar, rice, milk and grain cereals. That is largely the reason health food stores have sprung up not only in the United States but in many other countries as well. A recent visitor from West Germany told me that the German people have recently become highly enthused over health foods. They now have Health Practitioners in some cases replacing the medical doctors. The practitioners prescribe herbs and natural foods for staying well and for regaining health.

If you are overweight and want to become slim, change to a diet of strictly natural foods. Throw away the can opener and stop buying anything in bottles or cans. Remember, too, that even good, natural foods can be eaten in excess. Eat only enough to meet your bodily needs. Too many people eat mainly for the pleasure of eating.

Chapter Two

Reducing with Herbs
and Loving It

The high vitamin and mineral content of herbs is most helpful in their effect upon the body.

Dr. Bernard Jensen

HERBS provide the ideal way of reducing. In addition to making foods taste better, herbs are generally high in vitamin and mineral contents in purely natural form, easiest to digest and to become assimilated into the body structure.

LIGHT EATING AND HEAVY BENEFITS

The structure of the body can be compared to the structure of the airplane. An airplane is made of light but strong materials with the various wings and tail parts controlled by the pilot at a central control. Similarly, the human body should have a minimum of weight, sufficient to do the job of carrying the load. The body's nervous system, comparable to the wiring diagram of an airplane, centers in the brain under the control of you, the pilot.

What would you think of a pilot who selected oil and gas for his airplane on the basis of pretty coloring? Or a pilot who used cabin space for the storage of articles he did not need? This could be compared to eating fancy foods prettily packaged but not really designed to do the best job for the body's needs. Or it can be compared to the individual who eats or drinks more than what is needed.

Light but adequate eating should be the goal for all. Such a program brings heavy benefits. If you are healthy, it will keep you healthy; and if you are ill, the chances are good that it will restore your health.

COMBINING FOODS WITH HERBS AND SPICES

Some herbs and spices are more suited to some foods than to others. You do not just sprinkle any herb on any food. For example, sprinkling paprika and chopped parsley over potatoes is considered by many as an ideal combination.

Paprika is rich in vitamin C and for dieters who want to succeed in doing without sugar, paprika has the virtue of sweetening many dishes upon which it is used. It is often sprinkled on meat and fish dishes, eggs, sour cream and salad dressing.

A small twig of parsley is often placed on a dish as a sort of decoration and many people believe that it was never intended to be chewed and swallowed. Yet parsley is richly endowed with vitamins A,B and C and also has fairly large quantities of protein, calcium, iron, phosphorus and potassium. Copper and manganese are also present as well as some carbohydrates. Of 100 grams of parsley, 1 gram of it is fat.

Thus, you can see that herbs and spices do not merely flavor the food. They are themselves foods and are vital to your well-being. This cannot be said of either refined sugar or table salt. Neither sugar nor salt contains any food value in the form of useful vitamins or minerals.

Beware of herbs or spices that have been processed. A quantity of 100 grams of horseradish, for example, has 3.2 grams of protein in its raw state. This is reduced, for the same 100 gram quantity, to 1.3 grams when you buy it in a processed state, ready for market. Similarly, 100 grams of raw horseradish has 140 milligrams of calcium, but this is reduced to 61 milligrams after it is processed. The iron content is reduced from 1.4 milligrams to 0.9 milligrams and the amount of phosphorus is reduced to about one-half after processing.

The reduction in food value is bad enough; however, some manufacturers or distributors of foods add artificial colorings and flavors. Colorings and flavorings may not be harmful but they are suspected of containing carcinogenic (cancerous) substances and, of course, it is better to be safe than sorry.

There are numerous other herbs and spices used with foods that will be discussed from time to time in other portions of this book.

THE RELAXING HERBS
AND HOW TO USE THEM

Herb teas are an important part of any diet program in helping a dieter to overcome tension. Men and women sometimes become very nervous while dieting. Teas that relax the nerves and are especially suitable for drinking just before bedtime are bittersweet, bugleweed, passion flower and stramonium. There are a few others that have a relaxing effect but they are not mentioned here because, unless very carefully used, the relaxing effect is too strong.

Bittersweet is a climbing plant used for hedges. The twigs and bark of the root are steeped in hot water long enough for the water to absorb the taste and flavor of the herb. A slice of lemon should be added for taste and as this herb is slightly bitter you may want to add a teaspoonful or two of honey.

Bugleweed grows mostly in the eastern part of the United States. It has a mint-like odor but the taste is somewhat bitter and, again, some honey should be added to overcome the bitterness. It is always good practice to add some lemon to the tea. Prepare as directed for bittersweet.

Passion flower is also well known as a sedative tea drink. The plant and leaves are crushed and steeped in hot water to produce this relaxing drink. Incidentally, although its natural habitat is the tropics, it is being grown in greenhouses in northern climates. Its fruit is a large edible berry.

Stramonium is a European plant, the leaves and seeds of which are used to produce a relaxing tea. Dried leaves are crushed and placed into a teapot and hot water is poured over the leaves and allowed to steep for about ten minutes. Some lemon and honey should be added for flavoring. One-fourth to one-third of the cup should be filled with tea and the balance of the teacup filled with plain hot water.

Several relaxing teas have been mentioned as it may be difficult to locate all of the herbs. Any one of them would serve well as a relaxing tea.

HOW JOHN F. USED HERBS
AND SPICES FOR ENERGY NEEDS

You have learned about herbs that relax and now you will learn about herbs that give energy. The case of John F. is a good example.

John, 51, was of normal weight for his height after having recently undergone a closely supervised weight reduction program over a period of six months. However, he complained of a loss of energy.

On the theory that his reducing program might have resulted in an excessive reduction in nutritive food intake, I decided that he should try some nutritive herbs. In this way, he would get more energy without any danger of an increase in weight. There are many nutritive herbs, including arrowroot, Iceland moss, Irish moss, salep, saw palmetto and slippery elm.

John tried saw palmetto and slippery elm and obtained almost immediate beneficial results. The saw palmetto quickly restored his energy after two days of use. This herb is usually obtainable in a powder form made from the dried berries. Usually, the tip of the teaspoon is enough to hold a little of the powder with a cup of hot water.

Another nutritive herb used by John was slippery elm. The inner bark of the plant is finely powdered and is highly nutritious, being comparable to the nutritive value of oatmeal. A teaspoonful of the powder is placed in a teapot and a pint of hot water is poured over it. Some honey and lemon, cinnamon or nutmeg may be added to improve the taste.

HERBS AID DIGESTION

A good digestive system is important for the proper assimilation of food. Many herbal teas aid in digestion such as bayberry, bloodroot, centaury, gold thread, senega (snakeroot), and sweet flag (calamus).

For bayberry the dosage for tea is one teaspoon of the powdered bark to a pint of boiling water. It should be taken while warm. Take one teacup at bedtime.

Bloodroot tea is made by steeping a teaspoonful of the grated root in a pint of boiling water. A little of this root tea goes a long way. After the tea has soaked until it has cooled, take a teaspoonful at a time, six times a day.

The shredded centaury plant tea is prepared by measuring out a teaspoonful of the herb into a cup and adding a pint of boiling water. After steeping for about ten minutes, the tea is ready for drinking.

Gold thread is prepared as a tea by steeping one teaspoonful of the powdered root with a cup of boiling water for one-half hour and then straining it. One tablespoonful is taken three to six times a day. This herb tea is reported to be helpful in aiding digestion and it also improves the appetite.

Saw palmetto, also good for digestion, has previously been mentioned as one of the herbs used for energy. Many herbs have been found to have multiple functions.

The herb known as sweet flag or calamus is prepared by pouring a pint of boiling water over one ounce of the herb and allowing it to steep for at least ten minutes. After straining, (a customary practice after steeping any of the herbs unless the herb is in a tea bag) sip slowly throughout the day, one or two swallows at a time.

All the herbal teas mentioned are highly recommended for good digestion.

SOME HERBAL OILS FOR LOSING WEIGHT

Some experiments with plants have proved that many of them contain volatile oils containing a substance known as phytochinin, said to have an effect on carbohydrate metabolism. Keep in mind that carbohydrate foods are plant foods and that metabolism is a reference to cellular changes that take place in foods. By using plant oils found mainly in herbs, the improvement of cellular metabolism is likely to improve digestion. A more efficient digestion of food reduces the appetite for food that is not needed.

The olive is the fruit of an evergreen tree from warm regions of the earth such as the Mediterranean. The oil is commonly used as part of a salad dressing. A good combination is olive oil with lemon juice for mixing with lettuce, tomatoes and other ingredients of a salad.

Because of the ability of olive oil to act favorably upon the liver and the gall bladder, the use of this oil is highly recommended to prevent digestive problems.

Few activities are more satisfying than enjoying a relaxing tea after dinner. A few drops of the oil of wintergreen in a cup of hot water, with a slice of lemon and some honey, makes a fine tea for relaxing the nerves. This oil has long been known as a nerve relaxant. For anyone wanting to forget food and enjoy a good, healthy and relaxing drink, a tea made from oil of wintergreen is just the thing.

Eucalyptus oil is distilled from the eucalyptus tree leaves. Six to ten drops in a cup of hot water, with some lemon and honey, produce a spicy tea acknowledged by many as a preventative of many diseases and complaints. For persons on a diet who fear that dieting may make them sick, let them partake of some eucalyptus oil tea for insurance against illness.

The clove tree is an evergreen from the Spice Islands, north of Australia. Five to ten drops of the oil in a cup of hot water, with lemon and honey, make a stimulating tea. The digestion of food is improved and the food values are better utilized. Cloves have long been used to remove gas from the stomach and bowels. By helping digestion and removing gas, cloves are very helpful to anyone trying to lose weight.

USING ROOT HERBS IN FOOD PREPARATION

There are several dozen root herbs, including such well-known herbs as belladonna, comfrey, burdock, culver's root, dandelion root, ginger and ginseng.

There is little danger of herbs being used in an excessive amount. In the first place, they cost more in large quantities than other foods, and in the second place, the use of any herb in a large amount would have a taste so different from ordinary foods that the diner would very likely rebel at eating it. If the root of a particular herb is eaten in any amounts larger than a teaspoonful, there could be undesirable effects.

Let's discuss some herbs and explain how they could be used to your benefit. Belladonna has a root about three-quarters of an inch in diameter and about six inches long. Some of the benefits of this valuable herb can be imparted to your dinner. Cut off about one-half inch of the root and combine it with some other vegetable being served, such as mashed potatoes.

A characteristic of belladonna is that it increases the circulation. Increased circulation is especially of benefit to overweight persons because the functions of the body are all improved when the circulation is improved. After all, exercising, jogging and other forms of movement are indulged in for the purpose of stimulating the circulation. Some belladonna in the food will accomplish almost the same results.

The root of the comfrey plant is highly nutritious and richly endowed with protein and other important ingredients. For example, it is also rich with a natural form of calcium that is easily ingested into the body structure. The powdered comfrey root is often blended with unsweetened pineapple juice to make a healthy and nutritious snack between meals or it can also do good service as a luncheon meal without other foods.

Burdock has been reported as helpful in getting rid of fatty flesh. A little of the root of this herb can go a long way. Take about one-half ounce of the root, boil it with some potatoes and mash them together. In this way, you will give your family the benefit of the herb in what appears to be part of the regular meal. Beware, in mashing potatoes, that you do not use fattening butter or even sour cream as these dairy products really do increase weight. Use skimmed milk or low-fat milk for mashing potatoes. Spice the mashed potatoes with some paprika, mace and/or thyme for flavoring.

Culver's root is an herb long used for cleansing the bowels. At the start of a weight reduction program, this may be just the herb to use. Be sure to use a very small amount of this herb as a large amount may cause vomiting. It is best to obtain the dried root as the fresh root is rather strong in effect. For boiling with potatoes, use about one-half ounce of the herb to the pot of potatoes, for serving two people. Use a proportionate larger amount of the root for more people to serve.

Where reference is made to root herbs, it is not necessary to use the whole root. It is often easier to obtain the herb in powdered form from a health food store.

IDENTIFYING EDIBLE WEEDS
FOR USE AS FOOD FOR WEIGHT LOSS

A popular misconception about dieting is that it is expensive. This is not so! In fact, the opposite is true. If you are really interested in economizing, the truth is that the better the diet the lesser the cost.

For example, some of the best diet foods cost little or nothing. There are weeds growing in the fields, forests and along the road that are edible and that are ideal for weight loss.

One of the most common weeds is the dandelion, considered by many to be a worthless plant. Few people know that North American Indians have long used it as a valuable food and drink. The shiny green leaves are excellent as a vegetable for salads, containing vitamins A, B and C. For example, the vitamin A content of the dandelion leaf is more than five times the vitamin A content of an equivalent amount of lettuce or carrots.

The root of the dandelion, cut up and dried, makes an excellent coffee substitute. It is often roasted before hot water is poured over the roots to make some tea. A little lemon and perhaps some honey make the drink highly enjoyable. Dandelion root tea is an old-time favorite. The word *dandelion* means lion's tooth and is taken from the French language. It is so called because the toothed leaves of the plant resemble the teeth of the lion.

Dandelion roots should be dug either in the early spring or in the fall. If you want to imitate your ancestors, allow the roots to dry and then roast them in the oven. Put them into a grinder and the product may be used as a morning "coffee" or at any other time of the day. It tastes similar to coffee, looks like coffee but does not have any of the harmful caffeine contained in regular coffee. Dandelion roots are great for anyone trying to reduce because they stimulate activity of the stomach, liver, pancreas and spleen. They also tend to rid the body of accumulations of fluid in body tissues or cavities.

As dandelions contain natural nutritive salts, the leaves serve as an excellent salad when eaten green. Dandelion tea may serve as a cold drink during hot weather. The green leaves are placed into a teapot and boiling water is added to them. After steeping for about 30 minutes, allow the drink to cool in the refrigerator, strain and use as a refreshing cold drink.

For those who do not have the time or inclination to roast their own dandelion roots, the roasted root is available in health food stores.

The root of the ginger plant helps to remove gases from the stomach and intestinal tract. Use about one-quarter of a teaspoonful of the powdered root to a cup of warm water. If you have the root but not the powder, you can purchase an inexpensive small grinder that will powder the root for you. Or you can do what the old druggist used to do—pound the root until it becomes pulverized into a powder.

The root of the ginseng plant is highly esteemed throughout the world. Ginseng's power to stimulate secretory glands and organs make it valuable to overweight people. It is considered helpful in overcoming constipation, and thus aids loss of weight. What person can lose weight if constipated?

There is much controversy about the relative merits of foreign-grown and domestic-grown ginseng. After much study and research, I am convinced that there is little if any difference between home-grown and imported varieties. Ginseng is ginseng.

It is best to powder the root and sprinkle it onto foods, soups and salads, or make a tea out of it by putting about one-half teaspoon of the powder into a cup of boiling water. Add lemon and honey if you wish to make the ginseng tea more palatable.

WEIGHT LOSS AND MUCUS-FORMING FOODS

There is a school of thought with the idea that certain foods form mucus within the body, and that these foods should be avoided. A diet free of mucus-forming foods is considered healthy and good for losing weight. Perhaps you should take a good look at this type of diet, to see if all of it or a part of it might be suitable to your own condition.

According to the theory, certain foods produce a mucus substance in the digestive tract closely resembling paste or glue. Meats of all kinds and cow's milk, eggs and cereal products form this mucus. As a result, the stomach, intestines, kidneys, and other parts of the body are clogged, greatly interfering with the body's functions.

The mucus-free diet is one without meat, dairy products, or cereal-grain products, and must consist entirely of natural foods, unpasteurized, nonpreserved, free of pesticidal residues, uncooked, fully ripened, untreated and unprocessed.

Raw green-leaf vegetables and raw fruits are the ideal foods, according to the mucus-free diet program. This is recognized as the strict vegetarian diet, not having any dairy products.

Under this program, two meals a day are eaten, one in the mid-morning and the second one in the late afternoon. Liquids are not allowed with meals under this diet although tea or coffee is allowed a half hour after the meals.

If you try this diet program and feel that you must have lunch, you are allowed not more than a slice of toasted whole wheat bread and one baked or cooked vegetable such as cauliflower, beets, turnips or similar root vegetable. In addition, a combination salad may be prepared with such vegetables as raw grated carrots, cole slaw, or both. Depending upon what is available as fresh produce, you may have some cucumbers, lettuce, tomatoes or green onions. Instructions call for only one cucumber, one tomato, one leaf of lettuce or one green onion. Merely because the food is healthy and nourishing does not mean that you should overeat.

For dressing on the salad, use oil and lemon juice. Vinegar is out! Fats of any kind are unnatural and must be avoided. As a spread for bread, peanut butter is allowed or some other nut butter. When fresh vegetables are not available, canned vegetables are allowed to be used. Also, when fresh fruits are not on hand, dried fruits such as figs, prunes, dates or raisins may be eaten. Prunes are especially favored for keeping the bowels clear.

BALANCING ACID AND ALKALINE FOODS

Few people know that it is important to maintain a diet balanced fairly equally with acid and alkaline foods. This is also sometimes referred to as the acid-base balance. The reference to base is a chemical one; a base in chemistry is a compound that reacts with an acid to form a salt. Some base compounds are ammonia, calcium hydroxide and organic compounds such as the amines and alkaloids.

Amines are compounds that are the basic ingredients of proteins while alkaloids are organic compounds occurring in plants such as nicotine, atropine, morphine or quinine. Any compound that is base or alkaline will turn red litmus paper blue. Acid substances will turn blue litmus paper red.

Acid substances usually have a sour taste and are capable of neutralizing alkaline substances. Acids contain hydrogen. The chief acid forming elements in food are phosphorus, sulphur and chlorine.

It is essential that the blood and tissue fluids be slightly alkaline for the maintenance of good health. If there is an excess of acid, the condition known as acidosis exists.

Learn which foods are acid in nature and which foods are alkaline. Then try to have an equal amount of acid and alkaline foods, with perhaps more alkaline than acid. As a general rule, green leafy vegetables are alkaline, such as celery and lettuce. Other alkaline foods are alfalfa sprouts, asparagus, beets, cabbage, carrots, garlic, green beans, green peas, lima beans, mushrooms, onions, parsley, potatoes, pepper and squash, among others.

Acid foods are eggs, cheese, all meats, fish and fowl, nuts of all types, seeds such as sesame, sunflower or pumpkin, fruits such as cranberries, currants, blueberries, plums and dried fruits such as apples, pears, peaches, apricots, pineapple and prunes.

Dates, figs and raisins are alkaline and most of the herbal teas are of an alkaline nature, being mainly derived from green, leafy plants.

If you ever want to make certain whether a food is acid or alkaline, stop at the druggist and get some litmus paper. Ask for both the blue paper and the red. If you dip the red paper into an herbal tea or other liquid and it turns blue, you are dealing with an alkaline substance. If it stays red you are probably dealing with an acid substance. To be sure, try dipping some blue litmus paper into the liquid. If it turns the blue into red, you may be sure that you have an acid substance.

You may find it interesting to experiment with the litmus paper. As you drink various drinks, take out some red litmus paper and dip it into the liquid and see if it stays red or turns blue. If it stays red, it is probably acid and if it turns blue, it is likely to be alkaline. You can take an article of food, about enough to fit into the tip of a teaspoon, pour it into a cup and then add about one-quarter cup of water and mix it and make a solution. Then dip some litmus paper into the solution and see what happens. You can in this way determine whether the food is acid or alkaline. Remember that the objective is to balance your food intake rather evenly, with just a little more alkaline than acid.

HOW HELEN H. LEARNED ABOUT HERBS AND SPICES FOR WEIGHT LOSING

Helen H. is a friend of mine of long standing. When her husband was killed in an automobile accident, she began to ignore her own bodily requirements and allowed herself to get into bad eating habits. At only age 45, she began to put on weight that for her size, five feet, five inches, made her look more wide than tall. Her weight became 180 pounds, much too much for her height and for her health.

The loss of her husband seemed to take away Helen's interest in living. She was not suicidal but she simply could not take an interest in food or in her diet. It was when she dropped into a health food store and started glancing through the book display that she learned about herbs and spices. The book she noticed was my own *Modern Encyclopedia of Herbs* (Parker Publishing Company, Inc.) and the section that caught her attention dealt with the use of herbs and spices in preparing foods.

She learned the difference between an herb and a spice. (A spice is an herb with a fragrance.) She learned that alfalfa leaves are rich with minerals and vitamins; which spices to use to flavor soups, salads, meat and fish; names of delicious and harmless substitutes for coffee and tea; seeds to use in baking cookies, cakes, rolls and breads and herbs to use on appetizers.

She was eager to try out some of the herbs and spices from the wide assortment in the health food store (some general stores are also carrying herb and spice stocks) and started taking an interest in preparing appetizing foods.

Helen already had my other health book *Encyclopedia of Fruits, Vegetables, Nuts and Seeds for Healthful Living* (Parker Publishing Company, Inc.) and used it as a guide to make certain that she included all of the necessary vitamins and minerals in her daily food consumption. Within two weeks after picking up the herb and spice cookery, her spirits picked up and she was a different person. Helen eliminated the fatty foods from her diet (they did not go well with herbs and spices) and she started a weight losing program that gained her a sensible figure within 60 days.

ESTABLISHING REASONABLE AND SENSIBLE GOALS

A minister once told me that when asking for special favors from the Lord to ask only for small ones. "That way," he explained, "you are more likely to get what you want."

The same principle applies to weight goals. Aim for little achievements at first and the big ones will take care of themselves. Aim for a weight loss of three or four pounds a week. This is indeed only a small goal if you avoid fatty foods and substitute foods containing all of the necessary vitamins and minerals. A bonus to keep in mind is that you need not worry about the bodily needs for protein, carbohydrates and fats. Anyone who is careful enough to get all of the necessary vitamins and minerals daily from the foods ingested will be practically certain to automatically obtain sufficient protein foods, carbohydrates and fats.

The foods that contain vitamins and minerals also contain protein, carbohydrates and fats. For example, a serving of lettuce provides not only 22 milligrams of calcium as well as other minerals such as iron, phosphorus and potassium, but it also contains vitamins A, B and C as well as some carbohydrates and fats.

It is but a small goal, therefore, to be sure to have a serving of lettuce daily. You may want to substitute parsley for the lettuce once in a while or, better yet, have both of them. Parsley not only has all of the vitamins and minerals contained in lettuce but in addition has copper and manganese, two minerals that are also needed in the body—in a small amount, of course.

The point to keep in mind is that you take only one small step at a time. Resolve to include lettuce and parsley in your diet daily. This is not too severe a requirement and it gives you many vitamins and minerals, as well as protein and carbohydrates.

Include in your goal, at the start, a firm resolution to stay away from candy. After you lose the candy habit, resolve to stay away from ice cream; follow this up later by avoiding cookies made with sugar or containing preservatives. You can easily make oatmeal cookies and thereby avoid eating cookies, cakes and pies. Take some oatmeal, add an egg or two, some honey, a little salad oil and some raisins and you can bake a dozen or more large oatmeal cookies in just a short time.

Remember to take one step at a time. It may be too difficult for you to eliminate fatty and sugary foods overnight.

JOAN Y. FOUND PREGNANCY EASIER WITH HERBS AND LESS WEIGHT

Joan Y. was 30, overweight and pregnant. For most women, pregnancy is normally accompanied by a feeling of well-being and an excellent appetite. But not for Joan. Joan explained that it was difficult enough to guard against gaining weight during pregnancy without having to worry about getting rid of the extra weight existing at the time of conception. However, she knew that extra weight problem must be handled and without any delay.

When Joan consulted me, the first thing I had to do was to ascertain her diet. I had to learn what bad eating habits she had that brought about the excess weight. A program of food substitution would be necessary. Substitution is always better than elimination. A patient feels the doctor is trying to starve the patient to death if foods are labeled as forbidden and adequate substitutes are not suggested.

Joan was drinking too much milk, for one thing. Someone had told her or she had read someplace that everyone should drink a quart of milk a day and that's exactly what she was doing. Well, the milk just had to go. The butter-fat in her whole milk was simply building up her fat tissue excessively. As a substitute, I suggested two glasses of prune juice daily. This would clean out her system and get rid of her constipation problem.

I also told her that she would have to eliminate all sweets from her diet such as candy, ice cream, jellies, cookies, cake, donuts, carbonated beverages, sugar cereals or any foods with sugar in it. She did not need a case of diabetes when the time came for delivery of her child. The overweight, pregnant woman suffers from a very great strain on all organs of the body. Studies have shown that toxemia of pregnancy, a dreaded complication, does not affect women on nutritious diets.

As a substitute for sweets, Joan was advised to use herbs and spices in and on her foods and drinks. She was told to flavor her soups with allspice, thereby adding a flavor and delightful fragrance much more exciting than any sugar. Other herbs and spices used on soups are anise seeds, asafetida, basil, bay leaves, celery seeds, chervil, cumin, dill and fennel seeds, marjoram, oregano and tarragon. For a tea in lieu of coffee, alfalfa seeds or alfalfa leaves in hot water with a little lemon juice and perhaps a teaspoon of honey, not only adds vitamins and minerals to the diet but also satisfies the urge for something good to drink. This tea also happens to be highly nutritious.

Instead of white bread, rolls or biscuits made with white flour, I encouraged Joan to bake her own bread. A simple recipe calls for whole wheat flour, to which is added some water, salad oil and yeast. About one-half cup of the oil to about four cups of whole wheat flour would be about right. Directions for preparing the yeast are usually found on the package. Make the dough, let it rise for about 40 minutes, knead it, let it rise again, divide the dough into small biscuit sizes and bake in a moderate over (about 350°) for about one hour. Caraway or fennel seeds, or both, may be mixed in with the dough for flavoring. To make some excellent gingerbread cookies, take a portion of the dough, add honey to it for sweetening, sprinkle ginger into the dough and cut into cookie shapes before baking. After baking, you may want to sprinkle with cinnamon.

Joan was also instructed to have at least two servings of both raw and cooked vegetables daily, usually two for lunch and two for dinner. For breakfast, at least one egg daily, preferably two, as the egg yolks are superb for their vitamin and mineral contents. Lean meats should always be selected and emphasis should be on poultry and turkey rather than on pork or beef. Fish should be prominent on the menus but never any fried foods. When eating potatoes, Joan was warned about excessive flooding with butter.

With this program, Joan had plenty to eat and the benefit of an adequate supply of minerals and vitamins. The herbs and spices gave her food the tang she needed to make it interesting.

I explained to Joan that even though she should curtail her eating, her body required an adequate supply of protein, vitamins and minerals. Ideally, an adequate diet should be the rule even prior to pregnancy in order to prevent miscarriages and abortions. Pregnancy results in the need for more nutrients than normally required because of the growing fetus, with the need for more calcium, for example, for bone and teeth formation.

Studies indicate that the fetus stores iron for use during the first month of birth. Sources of iron include such beef organs as the liver, kidney, heart and tongue. Iron is also found in all lean meats, chicken, eggs, most green leaf vegetables, potatoes, dried fruits, dried peas and beans. I urged Joan to concentrate on getting her iron from these natural food sources.

To provide herself with an adequate supply of calcium, I urged Joan to bake old-fashioned corn bread, southern style, with whole-ground corn, also collard greens and beet leaves. Incidentally, beet greens are also rich in phosphorus, iron, sodium, potassium and vitamins A, B and C. Also rich in calcium are cheddar cheese and parmesan cheese, and they are also rich in phosphorus, sodium and vitamin A.

The result of all this was that within a month Joan's weight was down to normal and she was feeling fine. Her friends all admired her good looks, charming manner and happy outlook. Her baby daughter was born at home, using natural childbirth methods, and was a beautiful specimen of perfect humanity.

A SLIM FIGURE: THE KEY TO LONG LIFE

Your figure should generally be in proportion to your height, but an individual of a particular height may have a heavier frame than someone else of the same height. In such a case, the heavier-frame individual may weigh more than the medium- or light-frame individual. Correct weight, therefore, depends not only upon the age and height of a person but also upon the frame or build.

Many years ago, before much research was done, insurance companies prepared desirable height-weight tables based upon height alone. Later, they decided to show what the correct weight should be, depending upon whether the individual had a small, medium or large frame and also, whether the individual was a man or a woman.

For example, a woman with a small frame, five feet, seven inches high, age 25 or over, should weigh between 126 and 136 pounds, according to the tables. A man of that height and age, with a small frame, should weigh between 133 and 143 pounds, at least 7 pounds heavier. The same tables specify that a woman of a medium frame should weigh between 134 and 144 pounds and that a man of a medium frame should weight between 141 and 151 pounds. Where individuals have heavy frames, the weights should be about 8 pounds additional, for both men and women, the tables say.

A new principle or theory is now taking hold, based upon research indicating that after age 25 your body metabolism slows down at a rate of about 1 percent each year. As a result, not all the food ordinarily eaten during younger years is digested and transformed into energy in the process of being metabolized.

Your metabolism or degree of chemical change that takes place in the body's cells depends not only upon the food intake but also upon bodily activities. As you become older, activity usually reduces. Whereas in the past, the food-fuel was largely converted into energy and burned away, with only small amounts stored as body fat, as you get older more and more of the food is stored and the fat buildup may continue at an alarming rate. Habits of many years standing are often hard to change and a couple sitting down to eat a meal often find it difficult to reduce the amount of food consumed.

It is not surprising, therefore, to see people gaining weight as they become older, not realizing that reduced activity requires a reduction in food intake.

Studies indicate that after the age of 25 years, because of the reduction of body metabolism at the rate of 1 percent a year, the food intake should likewise be reduced at the same rate of 1 percent a year. Thus, starting at age 25, the food intake should be 25 percent less after 25 years. Few people realize this and continue to consume food at age 50 in the same amount as consumed at age 25 or 30.

Dieters should also know that sometimes the body metabolism is too slow because of an underactive thyroid gland. In many cases, the thyroid needs iodine in order to function normally, which in turn will help the body's metabolism. While iodized salt may provide the needed iodine, there is a tendency to consume too much salt, which has the unfortunate result of causing the body to retain water. By eliminating all salt from the diet, many people have substantially reduced the total body weight. A good substitute for salt is granular kelp, a natural salt substitute that is not only the best source of organic iodine but also contains calcium, potassium and various trace minerals. One teaspoonful of kelp a day, added to various foods and drinks, will provide a sufficient quantity of iodine to meet the needs of the body. The iodine stimulates the thyroid gland, which in turn stimulates the body's metabolism, which in turn transforms fatty foods into energy.

Chapter Three

Fitting Herbal
Weight Loss Plans
to Special Problems

It's supposed to be a professional secret but I'll tell you anyway. We doctors do nothing. We only help and encourage the doctor within.

Dr. Albert Schweitzer

EVERY person is different in many ways. Everyone is affected by their years of different food and drink habits; exercising or lack of exercise; different working environments and even by their years of growing up or adult living under different degrees of stress and worry. All these conditions have an effect upon an individual's special weight-losing problems.

SOME HERBS CONSIDERED IDEAL FOR SLIMMING DOWN

Every overweight person should be familiar with the names of herbs well known for use in reducing programs. However, as I have already pointed out, just as every person is different in many ways you must remember that the various herbs are also different in many ways. It is simply not practical to catalog the reducing herbs in one group and advise people to take those herbs.

In starting a reducing program, it is always advisable to first try to cleanse the system. There are special herbs for this purpose. There are also special herbs that reduce the excessive water content of the body, known as diuretic herbs. Other herbs stimulate various organs of the body to function better. Herbs that stimulate the liver and gall bladder help these organs to do a better job of removing toxic substances from food and drink. Other herbs are general stimulant herbs, stimulating the heart and muscles to normal functioning.

Another herb valuable in weight loss programs is alfalfa, especially in the form of alfalfa sprouts. It has been referred to as a wonder herb and the father of all foods. This is because it is believed to contain all of the known vitamins as well as many minerals, organic salts and eight of the essential enzymes. Alfalfa is rich in protein, providing the body with the amino acids needed for cell-building. The chlorophyll in alfalfa helps the body to resist infection.

As can be readily seen, the health-giving and protective properties of herbs are all-important to dieters wishing to lose weight without endangering themselves.

A common and highly dangerous method of weight-loss dieting is to go on a rigid fast or extremely low-calorie diet and combine such a regimen with vigorous exercise such as jogging. This often leads to heart attacks because the heart is overworked and the heart muscle is, at the same time, deprived of the nutrients it needs.

One of the important nutrients needed by the heart tissue is manganese, which is found in kelp, a sea-plant usually available only in the health food stores. This valuable herb, obtainable in dried, powdered form, should be placed into a salt shaker and used liberally for sprinkling on various foods. Kelp, because of its silicon content, is also known to keep the skin from wrinkling and to prevent hair from falling out. The calcium and sulphur in kelp are also helpful for preserving fingernails.

Alfalfa sprouts will provide the necessary vitamins and minerals needed by the heart and a gentle Swedish-type massage over the entire body will give the muscles and tissues the fresh supply of nutrients needed by the glands and organs, especially the heart.

If a good masseur or masseuse is not available and some mild form of exercise is chosen as an alternative, it may be a good idea to partake of the heart-tonic herb known as hawthorn berry. Not only is this herb heavily loaded with vitamin C, thus tending to prevent as well as relieve colds, but throughout Europe it is recognized as a very fine cardiac (heart) tonic.

Persons dieting are often given medication for reducing swollen tissues in the form of some kind of drug that has a diuretic effect, increasing the flow of urine by stimulation of the kidneys. The hawthorn berry herb has the additional characteristic of producing the diuretic effect.

It may be said, therefore, that the three herbs, kelp, alfalfa sprouts and hawthorn berries are ideal for the person wishing to reduce and to do it safely. There are of course many other fine herbs that can be used, which I will discuss later.

HOW HELEN G. USED A REDUCING CHART FOR PLANNED REDUCING

Helen G., aged 34, weighed 190 pounds and was only five feet, four inches tall. She was not only obese but had swollen ankles, flabby arms, legs like tree-trunks and a body entirely shapeless.

Under my diet programs, I insist that the patient obtain all of the necessary nutrients daily. No fad diets! So, to make sure that all of the nutrients are taken, I have a list prepared that I call my *planned reducing chart.* In the left column, I list all of the vitamins, minerals, enzymes and amino acids everyone should have daily. This includes carbohydrates and fat. The amino acids constitute the protein.

A new sheet is used daily. As the day goes on, the patient fills in on the right-hand side of the sheet the name of the food taken that supplies the listing at the left. It is like playing a game. The objective is to fill in all the spaces at the right side before the end of the day. If every space is filled in, the patient scores 100. Five points are deducted for every blank space. As the days pass, the patient soon learns how to earn a grade of 100 daily.

As in every other game, there are rules. The blank spaces must not contain certain words such as candy, cake, pie, cookies, soft drinks, foods containing sugar, white bread, white flour products, jellies, jams, jello or ice cream.

You can easily prepare this chart yourself. In your listing of vitamins on the left side of the table, be sure to include vitamins A, B-1 (thiamine), B-2 (riboflavin), B-3 (niacin), B-6 pyridoxine, B-12, B-15 (pangamic acid), B-17 (laetrile), C, D, E, K and P.

In listing minerals, include calcium, phosphorus, potassium, sodium, chlorine, iron, manganese, iodine, zinc, silicon, fluorine and copper. Some valuable minerals needed by the body in tiny amounts are molybdenum, selenium, lithium, vanadium and sulfur.

Also, the list should include folic acid, pantothenic acid, PABA (para-aminobenzoic acid), inositol, choline and biotin H.

In addition, do not omit including the bodily need for carbohydrates and a minimal amount of fat.

Enzymes should also be added to the list. Although produced in the human body, they are also produced by plants. Eating some live or raw plant food daily relieves the burden on the bodily production of enzymes.

Is the list too long? Do not fret. Just a few items of food, even eaten sparingly, will provide all of the necessary nutrition the body needs. For example, take kelp! Yes, take it daily! Try sprinkling some of it on foods. It is the richest source of organic iodine and many other minerals, including practically all of the so-called trace minerals needed in small quantities in the body, such as bismuth, chromium, erbium, iridium, lithium, neptunium, actinium, bromine, thalium and a few others.

By taking some kelp daily, you need have little concern about your body's mineral requirements. Kelp also contains protein, carbohydrates, some vitamin A and some vitamin B-2 (riboflavin) and vitamin B-3 (niacin). Because of the richness of kelp as a nutritive substance, it is especially valuable to persons who are unable, for one reason or another, to leave an inferior or deficient diet. Besides adding nutrients to food, kelp adds an attractive flavoring to dishes of all kinds, especially eggs.

Contrary to the beliefs of many persons having just a little knowledge, eggs are not harmful if not eaten in an excessive amount. An egg or two daily provides protein, lecithin (important for malnutrition and for breaking up fatty tissue), fluorine, iron, phosphorus, sulfur, niacin, vitamins A, B-1, B-2, B-3 (niacin), B-6 pyridoxine, B-12 (cobalimin), D, E, F (fatty acids), H (biotin), choline and pantothenic acid.

Thus by taking only two items daily, kelp and egg yolk, many of the blank spaces on the reducing chart are filled. Of course, there are still other blank spaces to be filled in. For many vitamin and mineral needs, have some green leaf plants daily such as a leaf or two of lettuce, parsley, spinach, beet greens, mustard greens, endive leaves, dandelion greens, turnip greens, cabbage or watercress. In addition to supplying many vitamins and minerals, they supply live enzymes.

Other foods that supply a large variety of healthful vitamins, minerals and proteins are brewer's yeast, whole grain cereals, including brown rice, barley, wheat germ and nuts, and legumes such as beans, lentils and peas.

Many readers already have as a reference book my previous health book *Encyclopedia of Fruits, Vegetables, Nuts and Seeds for Healthful Living*. This publication describes in detail the nutritive values of many foods and will be very helpful in maintaining the reducing chart.

To conclude the story of Helen G., I furnished her with a supply of 30 reducing charts, one for each day of the month. I asked her to indicate on the blank spaces at the right the foods she ate to meet the need for supplying the nutritive elements listed at the left of the sheet. For the first few days, her daily scores were extremely low. As she understood the program and started to change her way of living, she began to lose weight sharply and also began to feel better and have lots of energy. One of the things she did for energy was to eat two grapefruit daily, one in the morning and one in the afternoon while at work. In three months, Helen was down to a normal weight of 130 pounds, having lost 60 pounds in 90 days. The average daily weight loss was less than a pound a day but it was steady and she remained in good health throughout the program.

I should mention that Helen took a liking to alfalfa sprouts early in her dieting as I imposed no restrictions on the quantity of sprouts she could eat daily. She nibbled on them often during the day. There is a good deal of nutritive value in sprouts of all kinds and this did much to keep her in good health.

In listing the various vitamins to be taken daily, you may have noted that vitamin B-17 was listed. This is a reference to the vitamin known as laetrile, discovered by Dr. Ernst T. Krebs, Jr. This vitamin is found in such fruits as blackberry, boysenberry, cranberry, currant, elderberry, gooseberry, huckleberry, loganberry, mulberry, quince and raspberry, and in such seeds as buckwheat, millet, flax, apple, apricot, cherry, nectarine, peach, pear, plum, prune and squash. Advocates of the use of vitamin B-17 claim that it nourishes non-cancer cells and destroys cancer cells. The Food and Drug Administration claims that this vitamin is still unproven and that the claims have not been validated. Having met Dr. Krebs on several occasions and hearing him speak on the subject, I am convinced that vitamin B-17 is indeed worthwhile and that it will eventually become fully recognized.

HOW LAURA V. SLOWED DOWN
THE AGING PROCESS
WHILE DROPPING POUNDS

Laura V. was 48 and worried about her wrinkles, the loss of her hourglass figure, her graying hair and a frequent tired feeling. She weighed 190 pounds and, at a height of five foot, seven inches, was about 50 pounds overweight.

My routine procedure is to ascertain the kind of diet the patient is on. This gives me a pretty good idea of the nutrients missing and what foods are being ingested that really do more harm than good. I immediately noticed that missing from her diet were foods containing large supplies of vitamin A such as fruits, vegetables, nuts or seeds, liver, eggs, cheese, whole milk or butter. For breakfast, she would have some black coffee, followed by a candy bar, which would give her energy for a while and off to her job she would go. At 10 o'clock, it would be time for her coffee break and another candy bar. For lunch, she would have a hamburger and a coke, often followed by ice cream as dessert.

Her dinner menu would often consist of pizza, some fried chicken, a hot roast-beef sandwich, a corned-beef sandwich or a TV dinner from the frozen food section at the supermarket.

An evaluation of her food intake showed that she was lacking in several important and vital minerals and vitamins.

Skin problems, such as rashes, blackheads, wrinkles and related skin conditions are often the result of lack of pantothenic acid, a member of the B-vitamin family. It is found in royal jelly honey, human milk, egg yolk, wheat bran, brewer's yeast, broccoli, molasses, peanuts, liver, kidney and in nearly all vegetable tissues. Wrinkles in the skin are often due to the lack of nutritive elements required by body tissues, as is the case with most skin problems or, for that matter, many other bodily problems.

A tea made with dried comfrey leaves or powder, with some lemon juice and perhaps a little honey for sweetening, is highly preferred to cola drinks or even milk drinks. Cocaine usually found in cola drinks is a toxic alkaloid that stimulates the nervous system. It produces initial excitement and restlessness but is followed by profound depression, nausea and dizziness. There are cases where excessive cocaine has caused convulsions, collapse and death.

Laura was told to abstain entirely from cola drinks and to switch to lemonade made with honey for sweetening instead of sugar. She decided to take a thermos filled with lemonade and some ice cubes so that she would have a refreshing drink to take instead of coffee or cola. The caffeine in coffee causes palpitation of the heart, trembling, general depression, anxiety, insomnia and nervousness.

Laura's addiction to candy bars is typical of the widespread existence of "sugar slaves," people who are addicted to sugar. They enjoy that sweet taste and nothing you can do or say will dissuade them from enjoyment of that feeling of sweetness. Few sugar addicts known that the spurt of energy given them by a candy bar is not from the sugar but rather from the leaching effect of the molecules of this sweet-tasting carbohydrate. They travel through the body's blood stream gathering stores of vitamins and minerals from various body parts, where they are needed for tissue repairs and maintenance. Sugar itself is not a nutrient and has no food value whatsoever. The feeling of energy it gives is the result of a form of cannibalism, the individual gaining strength from a devouring by the sugar of nutritive elements already in the body.

After explaining all this to Laura, she promised to refrain from eating anything with sugar in it.

Despite general opinion to the contrary, milk contains a rich supply of sugar in the form of lactose or milk sugar. This sugar exists in milk even after cream is skimmed from the milk. Ice cream, a favorite food of Laura, is heavily loaded with fat as well as sugar and so is doubly dangerous. Laura promised to refrain from ice cream and to limit her milk intake drastically, using low-fat milk when possible.

I pointed out to Laura that recent governmental studies have confirmed what believers in natural foods have long feared—that the hamburger is dangerous. Aside from the question of vegetarianism, which is a subject unto itself, it is the intense heat of the grill or frying pan in contact with the meat that produces a carcinogenic substance or cause of cancer. The exact sequence is uncertain but my own theory is that the formation of cancerous cells is the natural result of the bodily mechanism's effort to remove foreign substances irritating tissues. The tissues are most sensitive to irritation when they are denied the nutritive elements required for optimum health.

Laura was cautioned not only to refrain from eating fried hamburgers but to also refrain from eating any fried foods, including fried fish or fried eggs.

For the first two weeks, I watched Laura carefully to make sure that she stayed away from the forbidden foods. I knew from my own personal experience the almost irresistible temptations to continue eating sweets, cakes, candies, cookies, ice cream and white flour products rather than whole wheat products.

I am certain that she did not immediately discontinue her bad eating and drinking habits but I realize that these things take time. As previously stated, there must be a transition period between the old way of living and the new; people cannot be expected to change overnight and to shed long-standing bad food habits and replace them instantly with good ones.

Within two weeks, however, Laura started to feel better and to lose weight. She began to lose some of that feeling of fatigue that usually beset her day and night. Actually, I think a lot of her fatigue was due to the energy wasted in carrying around those 50 pounds of surplus weight. It was like carrying around two suitcases, each weighing 25 pounds.

Her first loss of weight was tangible proof to Laura that the system worked. Weight loss continued steadily in the weeks that followed, with a regular loss of from three to five pounds each week. At the same time, there was no diminution of strength, and no weakness or inability to go about with daily tasks. Laura was indeed highly pleased with her results. She lost the entire 50 pounds of excessive fatty tissue within 12 weeks after starting her new regimen.

"I hope you're not going to make me stay on this diet forever," she said, "although now that I've grown used to it I suppose I ought to continue."

Laura had just stepped down from the scale as I was making a note of her weight. I wasn't quite certain whether she was really concerned about her diet program or wanted to know what would happen if she departed from the new health rules she had finally learned. I decided to be somewhat liberal.

"Laura," I said, "you have won the race and the prizes of good health and long life if you want them. There are many other invisible prizes such as the energy and vigor that will allow you to engage in your daily activities without having to take time off for visits to doctors and hospitals. You will save the expense of medications, X-rays and laboratory tests of all kinds because there will be nothing wrong with you, so long as you follow the health rules. An occasional deviation may not hurt you very much but keep it to a minimum."

HERBS THAT KEEP PEOPLE YOUNG

The herb that is universally acclaimed throughout the world as the panacea for all ailments and of greatest assistance for attaining a ripe old age is ginseng. It has been widely grown and used in Arkansas and other midwestern and southern states; there is evidence of its use by the North American Indians, and also in Europe and in the Orient.

The herb is largely used as a tea. About one-quarter teaspoon of the powdered root is placed in a cup and hot water poured over it. Some lemon juice is added, with perhaps a little honey and there you have it—ginseng tea!

Another herb of great value is cayenne or capsicum. It has several other names, such as African pepper, American pepper, chili pepper, red pepper and bird pepper. It acts as a heart tonic and gives renewed vigor to the body by increasing the circulation so as to improve the strength of the heart beat without increasing the rate of pulsation. It is used as a tea, placing about one-half a teaspoonful of the pepper into a cup and pouring boiling water over it. Some lemon and honey may be added to suit the taste. It should be taken when warm, one tablespoonful at a time.

Another plant of great value for maintaining youth and good health is rosemary. This is an excellent plant to cultivate in your garden or backyard because it usually grows wild in sandy and rocky places. It is fast becoming popular as a house plant as it grows well in containers and can be kept outside in good weather and moved indoors when the weather falls below freezing.

Both the leaves and flowers may be used either fresh or dry. It makes an excellent tea. Just place a few leaves in a cup and pour hot water over it. After steeping for a few minutes, it is ready to drink.

Rosemary is also popular when cooked with chicken, lamb, meat stews, soups and vegetables. The leaves may also be added to an omelet, for a special treat.

Rosemary serves as a heart tonic, it has a reputation for preventing baldness, quickening the mind and preventing memory loss, getting rid of excess weight, reducing high blood pressure and helping digestion and eyesight. If rosemary is helpful in even half of these conditions, it deserves the reputation of being a preserver of youthfulness.

These three herbs, ginseng, cayenne and rosemary, may not only be taken as herbal teas but they are also suitable as part of food preparations.

Ginseng has long been used by the Chinese not only for medicinal purposes but also for preventive or prophylactic reasons. Ginseng is easily powdered and then sprinkled onto foods of all kinds. It has also been made into an extract and the liquid mixed with various liquid drinks, all done as a precautionary measure to prevent the deterioration and the illnesses usually accompanying old age. There is no way of knowing for certain how effective ginseng has been but the fact that its use has endured for thousands of years should mean something.

Cayenne pepper, also known as capsicum, has food value as well as herbal tea value. Sprinkled on food such as eggs, it lends a pleasing tang to the taste buds and has the same general effect as the herbal tea, producing a natural warmth, improving the circulation and warding off the symptoms of colds, such as a running nose, sneezing and coughs.

Rosemary has long been a favorite among cooks for sprinkling over soups, meats and vegetables.

FROM CHUBBY SCHOOL TEACHER
TO SLIM, ATTRACTIVE WOMAN
IN SEVEN WEEKS

Kathy F. was only 32 when she started on my diet program. She had a small frame, was only five feet, four inches tall and weighed 165 pounds when she should have weighed not more than 120 pounds.

Kathy insisted that she ate very sparingly and could not understand her inability to lose weight. "After all," she pointed out, "I have only a cup of black coffee and a Danish for breakfast. That isn't much!"

I pointed out to her the dangers in both coffee and the sweet roll, loaded with sugar. The caffeine in the coffee was bad for her nerves, her kidneys and her heart, and the sugar in the sweet roll gave her only a temporary lift but actually was a drain upon her system and did more harm than good.

The white flour, used in making pastry, cakes, rolls and white bread is considered to be wholly without the vital ingredients found in baked goods made with whole wheat flour. Valuable minerals and vitamins are removed during the milling and processing of the whole wheat flour. Poisonous bleaching agents are used to make the flour look white and dangerous preservatives are added for a long shelf life. It can easily be concluded that white flour products are not only of little value but that they may also be quite harmful.

Kathy promised to avoid coffee and white flour products in the future.

For lunch, she would have a sandwich and a bowl of soup, usually followed by an ice cream dessert. Dinner usually consisted of steak and fried potatoes or some other meat with cooked vegetables, often accompanied by a fresh vegetable salad. Dessert would often be some rich pie, with coffee.

I told her the bowl of soup was fine but that should be the complete meal. I encouraged her to take with her to work about a teaspoon of brewer's yeast to mix into the bowl of soup at lunch. This would provide pantothenic acid and many other vitamins and minerals needed by the body.

As to steak and potatoes for dinner, with pie afterward, that, I told Kathy, would have to stop.

"While I don't believe it is necessary to count calories," I told her, "it is necessary to avoid fattening foods. The potato itself is a fine food, baked or boiled, but it loses its beneficial qualities when it is fried."

I explained to Kathy the great danger of mashing potatoes with cream or butter, making the mashed potato the cause of large weight increases.

I warned Kathy that some of the cattle raised in parts of the United States and the Soviet Union has been exposed to radioactive fall-out resulting from atomic bomb testing. In addition, many cattle are fed with weight-gaining chemicals prior to being transported to market.

Nearly all meat contains fat although most of the fat may be cut away before preparing it. Broiling a piece of meat seems to be the preferable method of preparation as this allows the fatty portions to drain away and the intense heat of the grill or fry pan to be avoided. Many nutritionists believe that the intense heat causes the production of toxic materials which are absorbed into the body when the fried or grilled meat is eaten.

The best cuts of meat are generously mottled with fat. This makes the meat more flavorful but adds greatly to the body's fat content.

While in beef, pork and poultry much of the fat may be cut away, this is not so with fish. Fish have fat distributed throughout the fiber and cannot be avoided.

Dr. Paul Bragg, a famous nutritionist and long-time associate of Bernarr Macfadden, known as the leader of the physical culture movement, advises users of animal protein to restrict this kind of intake to three times a week and to give preference to fish, organically raised poultry, veal, lamb, beef and pork, in that order.

Kathy liked chicken so she ate broiled chicken three times a week and substituted baked potatoes for the french-fried.

As for eating some pie for dessert, I persuaded Kathy to instead eat fresh fruit such as an apple, banana or mixture of cut-up orange slices, melons, berries in season or papaya.

She regularly included with her lunch and dinner some raw vegetable such as lettuce, tomato, cucumber, celery, onion or cabbage. For vegetables that needed tenderizing in order to be edible, I advised Kathy to buy a vegetable steamer. This is a small metal container that fits into a pot and prevents the vegetables from coming into contact with the bottom of the pot.

I also encouraged Kathy to season her vegetables with some of the spice mixtures on the market, which contain herbs of many varieties. They give food a new flavor and tang that will not only enhance the joy of eating but will pay big dividends in health and vitality.

Within seven weeks, Kathy had lowered her body weight to a normal 120 pounds. She also joined a health spa exercise class where she participated in group exercising and once a week allowed herself the luxury of a full body massage. Although a massage is often expensive, a good Swedish massage improves the circulation. When massaging is done around the joints of the fingers, toes, arms, knees, shoulders and hips many areas where blood has stagnated are refreshed with new blood which brings oxygen and nutrition

SHEDDING POUNDS WITH A COMMON ROOT HERB

The dandelion is widely distributed over most of the world and is considered largely to be a troublesome weed. The little yellow flowers can be seen everywhere

Although the dandelion is now widespread throughout the United States, no dandelion bloomed in America before the early settlers brought it to the colonies as a combination of food and medicine. Saturated with many vitamins and minerals, the dandelion plant was relied upon to ward off colds. Even the flowers were used, making wine from the blossoms.

The leaves of the dandelion plant are used as a salad and take the place of lettuce or other fresh greens commonly used in salads. The leaves can be dried and then put away for future use as a herbal tea or the leaves can be crushed and then powdered and used to sprinkle over soups and other food.

Dandelion roots are commonly roasted and then used as a coffee substitute. They taste remarkably similar to coffee and, of course, there is no caffeine in dandelion.

Being a mild diuretic, it is valuable in shedding pounds, hastening the elimination of fluids from the body and yet doing it in a harmless way without the numerous and dangerous side effects of drugs.

To use as a tea, cut the root into small pieces and measure a heaping teaspoonful of the root into a teapot. Pour a cup of boiling water over it and let it steep for about one-half hour. Use one teaspoonful for each cup of water. After it has cooled a bit, drink one or two cupfuls a day.

An interesting bit of information about the dandelion is that it contains more vitamin A than carrots and also contains vitamin B-1, known as thiamine, vitamin C and vitamin G, also known as vitamin B-2 or riboflavin.

Chapter Four

Overcoming
Slimming Obstacles

*Information based on experience is worth more than opinions founded on
theory.*

Dr. Henry Harrower

THIS chapter concentrates on the common obstacles met while coping with
the battle of the bulge. Practical solutions based on actual cases are usually
more valuable than theories that do not work.

THE SECRETARY WHO SLIMMED DOWN
WITH LIGHT LUNCHES

Mary L. had a problem.

"Doctor," she said to me, "My problem may seem to be foolish but I
think I'm overweight because of peer pressure."

"What do you mean?" I asked.

"I mean that I go to lunch with two or three other women in the office.
They all eat hearty lunches and when I hesitate about eating less than they
do they make unkind remarks and talk me out of eating a light lunch."

Mary was only 24 and weighed 140 pounds. This doesn't sound bad

71

but she had a small frame and was only five feet, two inches tall. Her weight should not have been over 110 pounds.

"Mary," I said, "you can eat just as much as anyone else, but just be selective in what you eat. For example, you might order a large fruit salad one day and a vegetable salad another day."

Most restaurants serve reasonably healthy salads at reasonable prices. Usually, the vegetable salad consists of a base of lettuce, with chunks of tomato, radishes, green peppers, some parsley and perhaps some slices of hard-boiled egg. Tuna fish salad also often includes all of these vegetables. This, and the egg, gives you the protein you need as well as numerous vitamins and minerals.

When eating a salad, avoid the dressings unless you want to use oil and vinegar. Also, avoid the white flour roll that most restaurants serve. If you have a strong craving for bread, ask for a slice of whole wheat bread, toasted. Toasted bread is easier to digest. You may spread just a tiny bit of butter on the bread, avoiding the margarine products.

I am opposed to margarine and prefer to use the animal fat, butter. From what I have been able to learn, in comparing butter with margarine, I know that artificial coloring is used to manufacture margarine and that the margarine itself is a highly processed product, much more so than unsalted, sweet butter. I have always favored being close to nature.

In any event, after Mary started having a fruit or vegetable salad as her lunch-time meal, she started losing weight at the rate of about a pound a week. In a few months, she brought her weight down to what was normal and, best of all, she kept it that way.

HOW EVELYN Y. USED HERBS
TO RETURN TO HER DIET PROGRAM

Evelyn Y.'s problem with dieting was that the food she was told to eat was not tasty.

"It's taking all the joy of living away from me," she complained. "I've got to quit it."

Evelyn really needed a good diet regimen. The motivation of reducing merely to look better or even to be healthier was not strong enough to justify giving up the joy of delicious and tasty food.

I told Evelyn she needed to put more spice in her life.

"Would it hurt your social life if you included garlic in your food recipes?" I asked.

"What social life? If I had to go out, a few mint leaves from my garden would cover up the odor," she replied.

I suggested to Evelyn that if she had not already acquired a taste for garlic that she should try hard to learn to like it. Garlic, I explained, is not only a seasoning but it is also a highly valuable, nutritious food. It contains a large amount of vitamin C and also has vitamin B-2 (riboflavin) and nicotinic acid, part of the vitamin B complex. Garlic also contains germanium, an oxygen carrier, which carries essential oxygen throughout the body and produces an invigorating result without side effects. Germanium has recently been mentioned as being an anti-cancer agent.

Raw garlic in large quantities can be harmful if you are in poor health. For example, anyone with a stomach ulcer should expect a painful reaction if raw garlic is ingested.

Garlic should be stored in a refrigerator to preserve its powers but not in the freezer. Keeping it in a deep freeze destroys the cellular structure.

Cooking garlic makes it lose most of its powerful odor and has little, if any, adverse effect upon the mucous membrane of the mouth or stomach. Even after cooking, garlic retains much of its nutritive value.

I also urged Evelyn to purchase a small container of mixed spices on the market to sprinkle over salads, soups and egg or meat and fish dishes. "After all," I explained, "America was discovered in 1492 because Columbus thought he was locating a new route to India, to purchase the herbs and spices of the Far East. Even in the 15th Century and much earlier than that, people were aware of the beneficial qualities of herbs and spices."

Evelyn was convinced and started using garlic and other spices and herbs with her special diet program. By thus being able to continue with her diet, she regained her youthful figure in just a few weeks, while enjoying her food and the good life.

MARY F. LEARNS AN EASY WAY TO COUNT CALORIES

Mary F.'s was the typical cry for help. "Dr. Kadans," she pleaded, "You have simply got to explain about calories to me. What are calories? Do

I need to count them up every time I eat something? Is there some easy way to count calories?"

After explaining calories to her, my answer to the next question was in the negative and to the following question I answered in the affirmative. Yes, there is an easy way to count calories.

The calorie is a measurement of heat or energy. The two terms mean practically the same thing. Technically, a calorie is the amount of heat necessary to raise the temperature of water from zero to one degree Centigrade. In the study of physics, the reference is to a gram calorie. In dietetics, the reference is to the kilogram-calorie or large calorie, a unit 1000 times as large as the gram calorie.

Is it necessary to count calories? If you know the rules and know what to eat or drink and what not to eat or drink and if you follow the rules, there is no need to calculate the calories for everything ingested.

Instead of counting calories, just remember to avoid the food and drinks that are deficient in nutritive qualities or that contain substances that may hurt you, such as food coloring, chemical preservatives, fattening foods, foods with sugar such as candy, cake, pies or sweet rolls, or drinks with alcohol, caffeine or cocaine.

Foods that are deficient in nutrition are simply waste foods, in more ways than one. They waste your money; they waste the valuable efforts of the organs of the body in the digestive processes, when these efforts could just as well be devoted to the digestion of better quality foods; they waste the space in your stomach and intestines, taking up space that should be used for the processing of pure and simple foods; they waste your time in purchasing such foods, waiting in line at the market to pay for them and wasting time preparing them and chewing them. They then waste away your heart in carrying the weight of these foods and waste the kidneys, skin and bowels in excreting them.

After explaining the two categories of food to avoid, the harmful foods and the waste foods, Mary was satisfied that she would not need to count calories.

"But, please, Dr. Kadans. Give me a few examples of waste foods. I understand pretty well that I must avoid food with preservatives, sugar, etc., but what are the waste foods?"

I explained that brown rice is more nutritious than white rice. The same applies to whole wheat bread as compared with white bread. Even though white bread is enriched, the pure and nutritious wheat germ and other vitamins have been removed and replaced with so-called "enriched vitamins" that are not natural to the product but have been artificially produced or synthesized in the laboratories. The synthetic vitamins are far inferior to the natural vitamins.

The famous nutritionist, the late Adelle Davis, once wrote that approximately 20 nutrients are milled out of white flour. She urged the purchase of whole-grain breads, made with stone-ground flour.

Other waste foods are the dry cereals so widely advertised in the media. Most of these cereals are contaminated with sugar (yes, contaminated) and much of the goodness removed, leaving only puffed remains of almost worthless food. An excellent breakfast cereal, on the other hand, is granola, consisting of wheat, wheat germ, oats, sesame seeds, honey, dried fruits and other natural ingredients. Anyone can buy these items separately and mix them together or the combined product is usually available in any health food store.

By avoiding the harmful foods and the waste foods and eating in moderation, enough to sustain and not to overload the body, Mary did not have to count calories and was able to overcome the calorie counting obstacle.

JOHN J. LEARNED
TO AVOID DINNER INVITATIONS

Invitations to dinner are mixed blessings. On the one hand, the food is free, the company is congenial and the taste is usually delicious. On the other hand, you eat too much, you gain weight, you endanger your health with food containing sugar, fat, salt, preservatives and perhaps many other harmful things.

John J. learned how to avoid dinner invitations by giving the stock reply of: "I already have plans for that evening." He might be planning to read a book or see a movie but anything is better than sitting down to a heavy meal that will overwork the digestive organs, add weight or clog the arteries with fat.

The hardest dinner invitation to decline is one from the boss. Could it involve a better position? Were you about to be appointed General Manager? Dare you refuse the invitation? This is indeed a difficult problem. Furthermore, the excuse of a prior engagement may not be adequate because another time may be selected.

When any invitation is received that is difficult to answer, fall back on the truth. Tell the boss, close relative or friend that you are on a rigid diet and that you would not want to ask anyone to prepare the kind of food that you eat or the kind of drink that you drink.

You may be surprised at the answer. You may be urged to reveal your diet, with a promise that this food will be prepared for you or, even more surprising, you may be told that you are not the only one on a diet and that the diet you are following is the very diet followed by your host or hostess.

HOW AND WHAT TO EAT IN RESTAURANTS

Another obstacle to following a diet is the necessity for considerable travel, with frequent visits to public restaurants.

Here, there are two alternatives. You may order selected food from the menu or ask the waitress if the cook will prepare special food for you to meet with the demands of your diet.

In selecting food and drink from the menu, it is often possible to obtain good nourishing food, without harmful substances, such as a salad with mixed vegetables or a fruit plate with fresh fruits in season. Another favorite dish for careful eaters is a tomato-lettuce sandwich on toasted whole wheat bread.

There are, of course, a variety of restaurants, ranging from the very bad to the very good. What you might order depends a good deal upon the kind of restaurant you are able to find or can afford to patronize.

I like to tell of the time when I had only fifty cents in my pocket, many years ago, before credit cards were in use. I entered the fancy dining room of the DuPont Hotel in Wilmington, Delaware and had a fine dinner for only fifty cents. I ordered a bowl of soup, which was on the menu for that amount and while waiting for the soup to be served a young lady was moving from table to table offering, without cost, from a cart, all kinds of raw vegetables such as sliced carrots, celery and cheese. I helped myself to an ample supply of these preliminary foods, partook of my soup and asked for the check.

You can see, then, that it is possible to eat at a fine establishment, where the food is fresh and nutritive, without great expense, if you are careful what you order.

Should you have no choice but to eat in a small roadside diner, where the owner never throws anything away no matter the condition, you can always resort to a tomato-lettuce sandwich, a glass of milk or canned tomato juice or other canned drink.

Although I stubbornly insist that canned foods are not as nourishing as natural foods and may even be dangerous because of preservatives added to them during processing, you cannot always partake of the ideal natural foods and have to deviate occasionally.

THE RETIREE WHO LEARNED
HOW TO STOP GAINING WEIGHT

One hears too often of retirees who leave this earth just a short time after retirement. What happens to them?

The cessation of early rising and off to work, with little time for food except for the evening dinner, results in an all day siesta of sedentary living with lots of fattening foods.

This is not the place to write about various retirement alternatives that will keep you busy, such as converting a hobby into a full-time business. I will assume that you have no alternative but to really and truly retire from all work of any kind. You are slim and want to remain slim but you have this obstacle of having lots of time and nothing to do with it. Consequently, you have the urge to spend more time eating and drinking.

The secret is to eat only those foods that will take up your time in preparation but are nonfattening. Nibble on carrots or on celery when you feel the need to nibble.

If you feel you want to drink, pour yourself a glass or two of skimmed milk on a hot day or some hot herbal tea on a cold day. On those hot days, you can take the hot herbal tea and let it cool and place it in the refrigerator to make a cool summer drink. It's easy to grow mint in your backyard. All you need to do is put a few mint leaves in some water, squeeze some lemon juice into it and you have a fine, wholesome drink.

If you feel tired and need some vitality, put a cup of yogurt in a blender, add a teaspoon of honey and a raw egg with half of a banana. This is a nonfattening drink that will really fire you up with vim and vigor.

Chapter Five

Nutrition Knowledge That Will Help Your Diet

The mechanism of the human body cannot be fully understood; it presents mysteries that baffle the most intelligent.

E. G. White

WE need to know more and more about the functioning of the human body. Much is already known but many mysteries remain. It has been said that the brain, in the digestion of food alone, consciously or unconsciously makes about 10,000 decisions a second. Simultaneously, decisions have to be made regarding the ingestion, distribution and metabolism of billions of molecules of food, the chemicals, enzymes or hormones to utilize for each different molecule; which to use and which to send on its way as useless waste; where to send the good molecules and where to send the bad; which juices to requisition from which of the glands, to help in the digestive processes as well as countless of other decisions to make.

No wonder, then, that we are advised to rest for a while after a meal, to allow time for digestion. Remember the old "safety first" warning not to go swimming for at least an hour or two after a meal? Give your digestive system a chance to function.

SETTING GOALS FOR WEEKLY WEIGHT LOSSES

It is a mistake to enter into a diet regimen that does not include all of the necessary vitamins, minerals, protein, fat and carbohydrates that the body needs every day. This is the only safe way to diet.

That is the reason I advise my patients to list all food and drink intake so that the two of us together can decide whether or not all of the required nutrients are being taken.

The goal set for any weekly weight loss depends upon the total weight sought to be lost, as well as certain other factors to be discussed. If the total weight to be lost is 20 pounds, this is a relatively small amount. A goal of from 1 to 2 pounds a week should be a sufficient rate of loss.

At the rate of 1 pound loss per week, it would take 20 weeks to lose 20 pounds. Two pounds lost per week would reach the 20 number in 10 weeks. The average (between 1 and 2 pounds a week) would be 15 weeks to lose 20 pounds.

One of the important factors to be considered in connection with weight loss is the physical condition of the patient. There may be some special condition to consider such as a weak heart, malfunctioning kidneys, damaged lungs, cirrhosis of the liver or other problems.

In such cases, it is most important that an individual establish a weight reducing program that does not conflict with the treatment of one's own state-licensed medical doctor. While it is true that the medical doctor may not be following the best method of treatment, many doctors having been sued for malpractice, the patient is obliged to follow the doctor's advice so long as the doctor-patient relationship continues.

The goal for the weekly weight loss, together with the contemplated weight reduction program, should therefore be submitted to the patient's doctor for approval when such patient is being treated for some medical condition, especially a condition affecting the internal organs or glands of the body.

To be sure you obtain all the necessary vitamins and minerals daily, it may be advisable to get some tablets or capsules that combine all minerals and vitamins into one tablet or capsule. Of course, the natural sources of vitamins and minerals are preferable, such as fruits and vegetables. However, it is often difficult to obtain all of the needed vitamins and minerals daily from the food and drink ingested, especially when you desire to severely limit intake of food and drink in order to have an effective weight reduction program.

There are also amino acid products on the market that contain all of the necessary protein requirements of the body. The use of amino acid preparations, together with the vitamin-mineral supplements, should be of great help to the patient desiring to achieve regular weekly weight losses.

Carbohydrates, another minimum requirement, are usually everywhere, especially in bread, potatoes and vegetables. The problem is usually in eating too many of them. A proper amount provides energy and heat; an excessive amount is stored in the body as fat.

While this discussion may lead to the view that most of the minimum daily requirements for vitamins, minerals, protein and carbohydrates may be met by merely taking one or two pills or tablets a day, unfortunately it does not work that way. The body is made so as to actually do the work of digestion. Just as a muscle atrophies if not used, so does the digestive system deteriorate if not used. The digestive system wants to work and needs to work. However, it does not need to be afflicted with having to cope with toxic substances because it will then break down. Natural and clean foods, free from preservatives and prepared in a wholesome manner—and not in excess quantity—are what the digestive system desires.

The weekly weight loss to be set is entirely up to you. Perhaps the greatest obstacle to be overcome is the habit of eating certain foods and partaking of certain drinks, usually in excessive quantities. Only you can tell the degree of willpower you have available to overcome those undesirable habits. If the willpower is strong, the goal for your weekly weight loss may be set higher, even as much as a pound a day.

However, should you feel a weakness in willpower and are unable to refrain from eating that hamburger, milkshake, cola drink, coffee, sweet roll, cake, white bread, canned foods, candy, ice cream or many other fattening and prohibited food and drink, your weight-loss goal should be set lower, perhaps a pound a week.

There is not much point in adopting a diet, failing to follow it and then blaming the diet for your own failure. Of course, this is not to say that every diet is good. If, after starting any diet, you believe that there is error in it, you have a duty to yourself and your family to protect your health and to discontinue the diet.

Unfortunately, you are often the victim of governmental uncertainty with respect to minimum daily requirements or the value of certain products. Perhaps the safest rule is to avoid including in the diet foods or drinks that are rated as unsafe by reliable authorities.

In setting the goals for weight loss, therefore, it is necessary to include in the daily regimen only food and drink that are generally regarded as safe and in minimum quantities. The weight loss will then take care of itself automatically.

HOW PETE C. SET UP WEEKLY WEIGHT LOSS GOALS

Pete C. weighed 230 pounds and was only five feet, seven inches tall. He was 49 years old at the start of his diet program. I told him that he was about 80 pounds overweight and he needed to cut out candy, cola drinks, coffee, ice cream, milk, canned foods, white flour breads, cakes and everything containing sugar.

I urged Pete to set a goal of losing 2 pounds a week. Under such a program, the weight loss of 80 pounds would take about 40 weeks.

We discussed the outwardly long time, 40 weeks, for reducing to a weight that would be acceptable to him as well as to any health authorities. Pete wanted to lose that 80 pounds within a month—4 weeks—rather than 40 weeks. I refused. I prefer that my patients lose weight gradually.

There are several benefits to a slow weight loss. One advantage is that it gives the nutritionist a chance to teach the patient the whys and wherefores of dieting—the functions of the digestive system—the food values and dangers of the various foods and drinks. I explain why it is not necessary to count calories; that, in fact, counting calories places a heavy burden upon the dieter—one that he or she is not likely to overcome. Perhaps that explains why so many weight-loss battles are lost. The chore of keeping track of calories is simply too much work—too time consuming and too tedious. Furthermore, it is unnecessary.

I said to Pete: "Avoid the fattening foods and your body will repay you with good health." I did insist, however, that he either take food supplements daily containing all of the vitamins and minerals or that he maintain the daily chart, already mentioned, listing all vitamins and minerals and making certain that food and drinks be taken sufficiently.

Pete soon saw that I was right. His weight loss was slow but regular. His daily weight loss was from one-quarter to one-half pound but all the while he was learning about dieting. We met twice a week for control discussions of his ability to maintain the program. By avoiding contaminated food and drink, his body tissues gained tone and strength and his metabolism improved. He was better able to digest properly the good food he ate. He began to feel better and to lose several aches and pains he had been starting to develop in his back, kidneys and other parts of his body.

Pete's weight loss goal of two pounds a week was met without difficulty. There was, most importantly, a slow conversion to a new way of life of a permanent and lasting nature. He not only gained his proper weight, with good health, but was able to maintain it with no difficulty.

THE NEED FOR ROUGHAGE IN THE DIET

Roughage is defined as the "indigestible fiber of fruits, vegetables and cereals which acts as a stimulant to aid intestinal peristalsis." A roughage diet has also been defined as a diet with large amounts of cellulose, water, mineral salts and vitamins. An alternative phrase for a roughage diet is a high residue diet.

In a normal condition of peristalsis, the food content in the stomach and in the intestinal tract, known as the alimentary canal, is propelled by successive movements of contraction and relaxation of circular muscles within the canal. The food content is first moved to the pylorus valve in the stomach and then to and through the colon.

Why the lesson in physiology? Adaptation to a good diet regimen must be preceded by an understanding of the functioning of the body. A good soldier is taught to obey blindly, without the need for explanations from his superior officer. However, a patient is not a soldier in the armed forces. In a free society, he does not have to obey his doctor and he can freely move to another doctor. But when the doctor explains the reasoning behind the directives, the patient is more inclined to follow the instructions received.

What are some of the roughage foods? The more common foods that provide roughage are leafy vegetables that are usually eaten raw, such as lettuce, celery, cabbage (shredded), parsley, beet and turnip leaves, etc.

A question often asked is: How much should the leaves be chewed before swallowing them? Another question: Is it all right to purée the leaves? To purée, of course, is to place the leaves in a blender with some liquid such as tomato juice and liquefy the leaves.

Chewing the leaves provides two benefits. First, the food mixes well with the salivary juices found in the mouth. Thorough mastication or chewing delivers to the stomach a product that is ready for the second phase of digestion by the juices of the stomach. These juices, called gastric juices (gaster is the Greek word for stomach), contain hydrochloric acid, rennin, pepsin, gastrin, mucin, phosphates, chlorides and other secretions, including at least one enzyme, lipase, which has the quality of releasing butyric fat from butter fat.

Slight chewing usually results in constipation. The famous nutritionist, Horace Fletcher, believed in chewing food until it simply disappeared from the mouth, entering the esophagus without any apparent swallowing action, or at least with a minimal amount of swallowing action.

By such thorough chewing, does this thereby destroy the value of the vegetable leaves as roughage? Not at all. There is still present, in the well-chewed leaves, the elements of the definition of roughage given earlier; namely, the presence of cellulose, water, mineral salts and vitamins. The cellulose fiber is not chemically changed or absorbed in digestion.

Other foods containing fiber include apples, apricots, asparagus, bran flakes, broccoli, mushrooms, oatmeal, onions, oranges, parsnips, prunes, spinach, wheat flakes, whole grains and whole wheat bread.

As to the effect of placing roughage food into a blender and liquefying it, the use of puréed food has both advantages and disadvantages. For those persons who have problems with their teeth and cannot chew well, the liquefying of vegetable leaves or other foods provides a means of ingesting food of this type whereas otherwise it would need to be omitted from the diet. It is also of value to someone too weak or too ill for the strength needed to chew food well.

The danger lies in swallowing puréed food too hastily. It is important to take a small amount in the mouth at a time, allowing the salivary juices to mix well with the food. The salivary glands produce ptyalin, an enzyme which breaks down the starches in various foods into simpler form. Another enzyme contained in the saliva is maltase, which splits maltose into dextrose. The saliva also contains mucin, which makes saliva viscid or sticky, and which also makes saliva a form of lubricant. There is also some thiocyanic acid in saliva, which gives saliva an antiseptic and antitoxic value as well as a trace of carbon dioxide. In solution, carbon dioxide forms a weak acid.

All of this explanation and discussion leads to the conclusion that it is vital to your well-being that food be thoroughly masticated before it is swallowed. If vegetables are puréed or liquefied, that is fine, but the product must be eaten very slowly and well mixed with salivary juices. Liquefying of food is no substitute for mastication.

MEASURING YOUR FOOD AND LIQUID INTAKE

While it is not necessary to keep a count of calories of the food you eat, including drinks, it is desirable to maintain some measurement of your food and liquid intake.

The basic rule to remember is that you are not to exceed one ordinary portion of each different dish. You may consider a fish or meat portion as one dish and two different vegetables as two additional dishes, for a total of three dishes. Some kind of dessert may be a fourth dish and allowing for one drink, preferably taken after eating the solid foods without any drinking. No meal should have more than four dishes and one drink.

For breakfast, usually three dishes and a drink would be sufficient. An omelet, two soft-boiled eggs or two poached eggs would be considered as one dish, some orange juice or half-grapefruit would be another dish and some cereal would be a third dish. A slice of toast would be another dish. For someone wishing to lose weight, the toast and the second egg should perhaps be omitted, depending upon the individual's height, weight and extent of physical activity during the day.

We have discussed the morning meal and the evening meal and now we will explain how to measure the luncheons. The meal with the maximum number of dishes is the evening meal with four dishes and one drink. Luncheon should not have more than three dishes and one drink. An example of three dishes would be (1) a portion of fish or meat, (2) a vegetable to accompany the fish or meat and (3) a slice of whole-wheat toasted bread. The drink could be a glass of buttermilk or some hot or cold herbal tea. The presence of some constipation might make it advisable for the drink to be a glass of prune juice.

For the serious dieter, dieting begins not at the table, nor when you buy foods at the market, but at your home or at your desk just prior to leaving for the market. At that time, you determine what it is you want to buy, make a list, and when you get to the store make sure you avoid all of the tempting foods and stick to your list. Avoid considering or even looking at other foods. When you see other food baskets loaded with those forbidden fruits, don't envy the buyers—pity them. Look them over, too. In many cases, you will see people who are grossly obese, who waddle as they walk. Unfortunately, they know not what they do.

Your measurement of your own intake becomes critical when you are making decisions as to how much food to prepare. As you place the portions in the pot, oven or broiler, keep in mind the number of persons to be served and the number of portions to be served to each person. In this way, as you measure out the food to be prepared, you are less likely to prepare more food than is needed. It is always best to prepare food fresh for each day rather than to eat leftovers or to offer them to members of your family. Reheating and reheating again and again is not conducive to healthy or interesting eating.

WHAT WILMA F. DID
TO PROVIDE PROTEIN FOR EACH MEAL

Wilma F. had a problem. She wanted to remain a vegetarian but was worried about getting enough protein with her food, a common problem among vegetarians and fruitarians.

"I'm not ill," Wilma said. "I am slightly under the normal weight for my age, height and build. My problem is lack of protein."

"Why do you think that is your problem?" I asked.

Wilma hesitated. I knew what she was thinking. Many vegetarians understand that there is but little protein in vegetables and restricting any diet to vegetables could be risky.

"It's because I feel tired all the time," she replied.

This made sense. Deficiency in protein can easily cause fatigue because proteins furnish heat and energy to the body and repair worn out or waste tissue. Protein also builds new tissue where needed. A feeling of fatigue is one of the indications of protein deficiency. I mentioned to her the thought that was in both our minds.

"I'm afraid that you're not getting enough protein in your diet because of your fascination with vegetarianism."

"Do you think I ought to stop being a vegetarian?"

"I'm not opposed to eating vegetables," I replied. "You know from the books that I have written that I have pointed out time and time again the many beneficial advantages of consumption of vegetables, especially of leafy vegetables."

"What can I do?"

"Would you be willing to eat an egg or two daily?"

"What if I did?"

"If you did," I answered, "you would be providing your body with all of the essential amino acids or proteins."

"Tell me more," she said.

"Eggs contain calcium, magnesium, potassium, sodium, phosphorus, chlorine, sulfur, iron and vitamins A, B, D and G. Eggs also contain lecithin, valuable for dissolving fats and helping to relieve atherosclerosis, the condition of fat clogging the arteries. Although it has been said that eggs should be avoided because they contain cholesterol, few people know that cholestorol is produced in the liver and that when diets are low in cholesterol the liver is thrown 'into a frenzy of cholesterol-producing activity, causing the amount in the blood to increase,' quoting the words of Adelle Davis in her book *Let's Get Well.*"

I also told Wilma that in order for her to obtain vitamin B-12 she should be sure to take yeast, wheat germ or soybeans. Adelle Davis points to documented research studies indicating that the deprivation of this vitamin causes sore mouths and tongues, menstrual disturbances and a variety of nervous disturbances. This vitamin, however, is also found in eggs.

The protein content of the egg was sufficient to warrant at least some departure from Wilma's strictly vegetarian diet.

"What about nuts and seeds?" she challenged. "This is part of the vegetarian diet and I eat them. Don't I get enough protein from them, as well as from beans and peas?"

"Almonds, Brazil nuts, filberts, pine nuts, pumpkin seeds and sunflower seeds are highly recommended. But you must remember that they are highly concentrated foods and so should be eaten sparingly. Also, they must be thoroughly chewed or ground in a grinder to ensure assimilation. Watch out for the high fat content of nuts and seeds."

"If you insist on avoiding eggs," I yielded, "be sure to include nuts and seeds in your diet daily."

Linda compromised. She ate one egg every other day and ate a serving of nuts or seeds or a combination daily. Within a few days, she felt fine and regained that energy and pep she had almost lost.

BUILDING NATURAL FOOD MENUS WITH HERBS

The most natural foods are fruits, vegetables, nuts and seeds. While the fruits, nuts and seeds are usually quite tasty without the need of additives, and while many of the vegetables have distinctive tastes and flavors that do not require any relishes or flavorings, a large number of vegetables seem to be tasteless and unappetizing without some spicing with fragrant herbs.

Remember that all spices are herbs but not all herbs are spices. The difference is that the herb with a fragrance is a spice; a herb without a fragrance is simply an herb.

Cloves are excellent for sprinkling over vegetables, especially over beets, tomatoes, potatoes and parsnips.

Chives, with their mild onion flavor, are frequently used in salads, mixed with the lettuce, tomatoes, green pepper, parsley, celery and other greens that usually make up a salad. Even when vegetables are on separate dishes and not part of a salad, chives are often sprinkled on the vegetables to give the food some tang, fragrance or flavor.

Cinnamon powder is popular for sprinkling over fruits as well as over milk drinks, puddings, pies and other desserts.

If on some cold day, you should decide to make a hot vegetable soup, sprinkle into the soup some allspice or some other spicy herb such as anise, asafetida, basil, bay leaves, cayenne, celery seeds, chervil, cumin seeds, dill seeds, fennel seeds, garden burnet, garden marjoram, garlic powder, ginger, mace, oregano, paprika, pepper, rosemary, tarragon and thyme.

Mace is a spice from the nutmeg tree and is used to add flavor to such vegetables as carrots, cauliflower, squash, swiss chard, spinach and potatoes, especially if they are mashed or creamed. Mace adds much to the flavor of cooked apples, cherries, prunes and apricots and has already been mentioned as a flavoring for soups.

Nutmeg may be used to add flavoring over all foods where mace is used.

Despite the fact that medical science has long ago invalidated the notion that spices may be dangerous to persons on special diets such as the so-called bland diet for ulcer sufferers, there are still many medical doctors who are either unaware of these scientific advances or who prescribe bland diets because their patients expect them to do so. They therefore tell their patients to go on bland diets. However, the latest scientific information is to the contrary.

Now that you know which herbs to use for various foods, let's discuss a few natural food menus. For example, what herbs could you use for breakfast?

The "good old-fashioned" country breakfast was loaded with calories. It would start with some orange juice, followed by a large bowl of some porridge such as oatmeal, cornmeal or other grain. The main course would then follow, which would be either bacon and eggs, ham and eggs or sausage and eggs, with hot biscuits or pancakes and lots of butter, with coffee or cocoa. There would be plenty of milk or cream for the porridge and the coffee. Sugar would be sprinkled over the porridge and often some sugar added to the drink.

Such a breakfast alone would add up to approximately 1800 calories and this was just the starter for the day. Counting the various portions of food for the breakfast described, there would be five "dishes" and one drink. The fruit juice at the start would not be counted as a drink but as a dish.

Obviously, starting the day with a breakfast of 1800 calories does not lead to any reduction of weight. Two or three dishes and a drink would be sufficient.

One dish would be an orange or two—not only the juice, but the pulp as well. The orange gives you vitamins A, B-1, B-2, B-3, C, protein, fat, carbohydrates, calcium, iron, phosphorus, potassium, magnesium, sodium, chlorine and sulfur. With all of these elements, oranges have earned the reputation for relieving hunger pangs.

Orange peel is a fine candy substitute for children or adults. Cut the peel into strips about one-quarter inch wide and boil for about 15 minutes with a teaspoon of salt. Then, pour out the water, add fresh water without the salt and boil again for 15 minutes. Pour out and boil a third time for 15 minutes without the salt. Allow the strips to drain thoroughly, dip into honey and they will be ready to serve.

Incidentally, for persons wishing to avoid that regular nightcap, a drink of orange juice will usually cause the thirst for alcohol to disappear.

A dash of mace sprinkled over orange sections or juice adds an intriguing taste to the orange. Some other spices that may be used for flavoring the orange are cinnamon, clove, allspice and ginger. They may be used separately or in combination with one another, as may best suit the taste.

Mace is the protective shell or cover of the nutmeg kernel. The nutmeg is processed separately and the covering is separated, dried and ground into what is known as mace. As mentioned, mace is fine for sprinkling over various vegetables.

A second dish for breakfast would be an egg or two, depending upon the activity of the individual. One living a rather sedentary life, with hardly any bodily movement, may do well to limit the ingestion of the wealth of vitamins and minerals found in the egg to one a day. Others may take two a day for breakfast, which I have done throughout my lifetime. Eggs may also be sprinkled with the spices mentioned for use with the orange or for orange juice. Cayenne pepper is also popular for sprinkling over eggs.

As a natural food, fresh eggs from healthy hens may be eaten raw. However, an egg boiled for three minutes is often preferred by many.

With the orange as one dish, the eggs as another, the third dish may be a slice of toasted whole wheat bread, with a light coating of sweet, unsalted butter. Toasting bread makes it easier to digest. If you do not have the time to bake your own bread, using pure whole wheat flour, be sure to watch the labels when you go to the store to purchase bread. Avoid bread with preservatives, sugar, chemicals or bleached flour.

As previously mentioned, butter is preferable to margarine. First, margarine has had coloring added to it and all coloring is suspect in view of recent findings that cancer may be caused by food coloring. Second, there is the question of rancidity or staleness of the margarine. It has been reliably reported that substances are used to hide the odors of rancid margarine but this covering of the odor does not eliminate the dangerous effects of using rancid or stale food products. Should fresh butter, unsalted, become rancid, its change in color, smell and taste is easily noticed and it may then be discarded.

For dieters who really want to reduce in earnest and get quick results, there is what is known as the monotrophic meal, a program of natural food eating devised by Dr. Elizabeth McCarter with her husband, Dr. Robert W. McCarter, outstanding and nationally known nutrition researchers, writers and lecturers.

The McCarters explain that mono means single and that trophic pertains to food. For breakfast, a diet of only one food is allowed, such as oranges, soaked figs, ripe peaches, soaked prunes, watermelon or other fruit. The dieter may eat as much of the single food as desired. As a rule, there will not be any excessive eating because there will be no aromas or sights of other foods in the vicinity to inflame the appetite.

The ideal natural food lunch, as recommended by the McCarters, would be a choice of baked potatoes, very ripe bananas, boiled or baked rice, or not over one-quarter cup of almonds or Brazil nuts. The evening meal would be a choice of tomatoes, plain lettuce, grated carrots, raw applesauce or alfalfa sprouts.

The matter of drinking with meals deserves some special attention. Buttermilk is a fairly good drink. In addition to some fat content, it contains protein, carbohydrates, calcium, magnesium, potassium, sodium, phosphorus, chlorine, iron and vitamins A, B, C and G. It is generally easily digested and provides the body with numerous nutrients.

Another popular drink among those wishing to live long and healthfully is grapefruit juice. It contains protein, fat, carbohydrates, calcium, magnesium, potassium, sodium, phosphorus, chlorine, sulfur, iron, vitamins A, B, C and G. Grapefruit juice is especially favored as a drink that may be taken frequently during the day to give you some energy, without having to eat a candy bar, coffee or an alcoholic drink to get enlivened. For those wishing to break from the tobacco habit, a drink of grapefruit juice instead of smoking a cigarette may be helpful.

Natural food menus for evening meals should be kept simple. People often mistakenly believe that large amounts of protein are needed daily and it is difficult to change habits of many years of indulgence in meat, fish, poultry, milk and cheeses. In addition to one or two eggs for breakfast, eggs are hard-boiled and sent along with lunch bags or included into custards and other dishes. Some estimates indicate that perhaps twenty times the needed amount of protein is ingested daily by millions of people. This is great for the meat and dairy industries but difficult for the digestive system.

Excessive food, especially protein foods, overloads the kidneys and liver and stimulates metabolism. Studies have shown, for example, that tribes eating large quantities of meat have short life spans and they become more susceptible to degenerative and infectious diseases, including rheumatism, neuritis, sciatica, nephritis and various liver diseases.

An example of a simple natural food dinner would be a baked yam, some romaine lettuce, alfalfa sprouts and a cucumber.

Despite much talk to the contrary, researchers have found that the average person, even a growing child, does not need more than one and one-half ounces of protein daily. Unfortunately, too many people think that they must have a half-pound hamburger or a steak weighing at least three-quarters of a pound, in order to meet the daily protein needs.

Actually, the requirements of protein can be met by ingesting one-quarter cup of nuts or two tablespoonfuls of pumpkin or sunflower seeds.

It is not necessary to refrain entirely from eating meat, although many vegetarians manage nicely without animal products. However, when you do eat meat, fish or poultry be sure to include an ample supply of leafy vegetables in order to obtain the minerals and the alkalinity of fresh, leafy vegetables.

In addition to alfalfa sprouts, other sprouts may be tried occasionally such as mung bean sprouts or wheat grass, from the sprouting of wheat.

HOW ROBERT B. RID HIMSELF OF HIS PAUNCH

"Doc, what can you do about this paunch?" Robert B. asked.

Robert was 39 years old, held a sedentary supervisory position and weighed 220 pounds. His height was five feet, eleven inches, with a medium frame and his weight should not have been more than 165 pounds, making him 55 pounds overweight.

I hesitated in placing Robert on a natural food diet immediately. Of course, it would have done him a lot of good but he would undoubtedly consider it as a temporary measure and as soon as his weight was reduced to a normal weight he would soon return to the same lifestyle that brought about the excess weight in the first place. No, I would have to go the slow and sure way.

"What have you been eating, Robert?"

Robert's reply was typical. He had been overeating, of course. Not only did he overeat but his wife and children overate too. So did his parents and his wife's parents. It was indeed a way of life.

"Robert," I said, "I'm not going to ask you to make any radical change in your diet because even if you followed my instructions and lost a lot of weight, you would not understand the reasoning or rationale behind the whole program. Instead, I'm going to start out by asking you to reduce by one-half everything you would ordinarily eat. Instead of two slices of bread, eat one. Instead of two eggs for breakfast, eat one. Do the same with everything."

I then explained to Robert the minimum requirements of the body for various vitamins and minerals as well as for protein, carbohydrates and some fat. I didn't explain it all at one time, only the fundamentals and very briefly. There is a limited attention span for everyone.

After a week, Robert came in again. This time I started explaining to him about the dangers of certain foods he had on his diet list, especially the large amount of canned foods his family ate, telling him that fresh foods were much healthier. I pointed out the need for some leafy vegetables daily, to get the minerals and the live enzymes they contain. Cooked or canned foods are heated to the point that all life in the foods is destroyed. I gave him a little lecture about the results of eating dead foods, how the enzyme-producing glands of the body are overworked producing enzymes needed for digestion and this causes them to age rapidly and wear out.

As time went on, Robert learned about diet and nutrition. He became very cooperative and actually changed his style of living. He also convinced his wife and between the two of them they were able to change the eating habits of their children, who had been fast becoming little fatties.

Within two months, Robert had rid himself of his paunch and, best of all, he had learned about nutrition and the necessity for proper dieting.

WHY NATURAL FOODS ARE BEST FOR YOU

When the Lord made the human body, He intended it to function along certain basic lines. Ideally, the body is designed to handle plain foods, in fresh condition and of sufficient variety so as to provide all of the necessary nutrients.

There are all kinds of fruits, vegetables, nuts, seeds and grains (although grains are really seeds of a plant) sufficient to provide all of the nutritional needs of the body. Trouble develops when these foods are transformed from their natural products, as a result of so-called processing, into articles that are more or less dangerous.

One of the principal food hazards is the presence of preservatives in food, which are used to lengthen the shelf life of various products for economic reasons. Advocates of the long shelf life and the use of preservatives claim that because of the many millions of mouths that need to be fed daily it would be impossible to bring fresh foods to the markets on time.

In order to obtain the natural foods that are best for you, you must either grow fruits and vegetables or locate sources for the purchase of natural foods. A disadvantage in buying from food markets is that as a rule the fruits and vegetables have been sprayed with insecticides while growing to prevent the insects from devouring them before they are harvested. Insecticides are known to damage the bone marrow.

Because of concern about the widespread use of insecticides among commercial farmers, many small farmers have established insecticide-free farming methods. Not only have they learned to farm without the use of insecticides but they have also learned to farm without the use of chemical fertilizers, confining themselves to the use of horse or cattle manure or chicken droppings. Often, a crop, instead of being harvested, will be plowed into the soil to return the nutrients contained in the crop to the soil.

It is already well established that various chemicals in foods, either as additives to preserve or color them, or as the remains of pesticides, are related to the onset of cancer. In experiments with small animals, it has been found that a diet of natural foods protects them from cancer. This was verified as far back as 1951 in an article in *Cancer Research*, volume 11, page 180.

The various combinations of nutrients in natural foods defy scientific analysis. Just as the contents and effects of various herbs are little understood by the scientific community, there is only a limited understanding of the effects of the various fruits and vegetables upon the body. It is possible to evaluate the quantity of vitamins and minerals of most foods but there is only limited knowledge of the quality of these minerals and vitamins. Of much significance is the stage at which the food is eaten. A banana with dark spots on the skin is more easily digested because it indicates that the starch in the banana has been converted into a completely digestible fruit sugar.

In many cases, the best parts of a natural food are discarded. For example, the skin of the peach contains more vitamins than the remainder of the fruit. Of course, the fuzzy part of the skin should be removed. Peaches are high in vitamins A and C and have an alkaline reaction in the digestive system despite containing malic, tartaric and citric acid.

The skin of the potato likewise contains valuable minerals and vitamins and is considered by nutritionists to be the most valuable part of the potato. The protein content of the potato is extremely high, although small in quantity. It has been reported that all of the essential amino acids (protein elements) are contained in the potato, which definitely places it in the category of a health food.

One ripe bell pepper may contain as many as 300 milligrams of vitamin C, whereas the average orange contains only about 50 milligrams. Although the bell pepper is usually seen in the markets as a red pepper, it is edible while it is still green and even before it has reached its maximum growth. Actually, it is not truly ripe until it turns red. When sliced and mixed with sliced or cut-up carrots, radishes and celery, a pepper can make a fine-tasting salad.

With the exception of parsley, cabbage is the best source of vitamin C. Cabbage, as well as the other vegetables heretofore mentioned, except for the potato, can and should be eaten raw, preferably as soon after being picked as possible. Cabbage should not be shredded until ready to be eaten. Ample amounts of cabbage juice are reputed to relieve ulcers. The anti-ulcer factor in cabbage has been identified as vitamin U.

There are innumerable combinations of fruit salads and vegetable salads, limited only by the imagination and whatever produce is in season and available.

Aside from salads, there is the mono-melon diet. This is eating only one kind of a melon for the entire meal, whether it be watermelon, cantaloupe, casabas or other varieties. Melons are especially valuable for kidney problems because of the diuretic effect. The mono-grape diet is similar. Grapes of every variety, taken in a meal without any other food, have a cleansing effect and are also known to help reestablish the acid-alkaline balance in the body.

Dr. N.W. Walker, a famous nutritionist, writes of the great value of grapefruit, in its unprocessed natural form, as a highly beneficial natural food helpful in removing or dissolving inorganic calcium, which may have formed deposits in the joints. The natural product has organic salicylic acid, not found in canned grapefruit juice, and it is this acid which helps the joint cartilages, removing the calcium deposits that have formed there, usually due to ingestion of devitalized white flour products.

The two key words to remember are *natural* and *raw*. Natural, when produced with natural fertilizers rather than chemical and free from preservatives, is used by food processors for long shelf life. Raw, because cooking destroys the life in food. Cooked food leaves a coating of slime throughout the intestinal tract, whereas well-chewed natural foods, mixed with salivary and gastric juices, without any toxic additives, move through the digestive organs easily and are readily absorbed by the blood circulation system for distribution throughout all cells and parts of the body.

PATRICIA B. DECIDES TO RESTRICT HERSELF TO UNCOOKED FOODS

Patricia B. was truly frustrated.

"I've tried everything," she told me. "I'm 40, fat and probably foolish. I'm only five feet, five inches tall and my weight should be not more than 130 pounds, yet I weigh 165 pounds. I have a medium frame and I'm at least 35 pounds overweight. I don't know what to do about it."

"You say you've tried everything. Have you tried a diet of uncooked, natural foods?"

"Are you saying that foods can be eaten without having to cook them?" she asked. I could see I had her attention and that she was waiting anxiously for my reply.

"Of course, they can," I answered. I told her of the many advantages of natural foods; how the enzymes in live plants help in the digestion of foods; and pointed out that the body requires the furnishing of the requisite 40 nutrients that the body cannot produce itself, namely, 15 vitamins, 14 minerals, 10 amino acids and 1 essential fatty acid.

"The body cares not at all," I explained, "whether the nutrients are received hot or cold, cooked or uncooked, so long as they arrive in good condition and of high quality."

Patricia decided to restrict herself to uncooked foods and to see what happens. She admitted that she had reservations. Would the food taste good? Would it be hard to chew? Would it be expensive? Would it be readily available? Would she know how to prepare it and which combinations of food to use? Would she have to purchase some expensive food processing appliances?

I assured Patricia that she need have no fears and that all of her doubts would be resolved favorably.

Taking up her doubts one at a time, I asked her to start with a variety juice cocktail for breakfast the next morning.

"But what will I do with the eggs, bread, butter, bacon, fish and all the other foods I have that are not strictly natural foods? The cost of food is so high that I just hate to throw all that expensive food away," she said.

I had the feeling that if I argued with her on this point, there would be no natural foods regimen at all. Better later than never.

"All right now, the next time you go to market, buy celery, water-promise me that from now on you will buy only strictly natural foods."

"Okay. I'll do it," she promised.

"All right now, the next time you go to the market, buy celery, watercress, two cucumbers, three or four tomatoes and a small package of parsley. Make a juice cocktail for your breakfast the next day after you make these purchases and that will be all you will have for your breakfast. If you do not already have a juicer to make juice out of fruits and vegetables, you had better get one right away. There are some inexpensive food processors on the market now that will juice, shred or slice fruits and vegetables. It will make them so appetizing you will wonder how you were able to get along without one."

In telling all this to Patricia, I was not exaggerating. For years, I have experienced the benefits and pleasures of using blenders, juicers and various other kinds of fruit and vegetable processors. The food actually tastes better when sliced or shredded, made into juice or blended with other fruits or vegetables.

"How much of this breakfast cocktail should I drink?" she asked.

"I suggest you make about two ounces each of the celery juice, cucumber juice and watercress juice, three ounces of the tomato juice and one ounce of the parsley juice. This makes a total of ten ounces, which should be enough for your breakfast," I replied.

She was concerned whether or not this would taste good. I assured her this would be a very tasty and delicious drink. There would be no problem in chewing it; in fact, it should be swallowed in dribs and drabs so that the salivary juices in the mouth would have a chance to mingle with the juices and prepare them for the stomach.

As to the nourishment in the breakfast cocktail, I pointed out that celery contains vitamins B and C as well as protein, fat, carbohydrates, calcium, iron, phosphorus and potassium; that cucumbers have vitamins A, B and C, as well as protein, fat, carbohydrates, calcium, iron, phosphorus and potassium; that watercress not only contains vitamins A, B and C but also vitamins E and G as well as protein, fat, carbohydrates, calcium, iron and phosphorus; that tomatoes not only contain vitamins A, B and C but also vitamin K, as well as protein, calcium, iron, phosphorus and potassium; and, finally, that parsley contains not only vitamins A, B and C but also protein, fat, carbohydrates, calcium, iron, phosphorus, potassium, copper and manganese.

"But, Dr. Kadans," she exclaimed. "What would people say if I told them that instead of the regular breakfast foods of eggs, toast, cereals, orange juice and coffee, I drank vegetable juices instead? They would laugh at me."

I was a little taken back by this protest. It's hard enough getting people to get onto a natural foods program. But it's doubly hard when dealing with people who fear criticism or laughter from their peers, friends and family members.

"Please, Patricia," I pleaded. "There is no law that says that you have to drink orange juice and coffee, and eat eggs, cereal and toast for breakfast. Your body just needs nourishment."

I told Patricia that the combinations of fruits and vegetables for anyone wishing to go on a natural foods diet program are simply endless and that these combinations can be prepared in such manner that they would delight and please much more than any cooked meal.

I told her of a delicious fruit cake recipe made with raisins, figs, dates, prunes and coconut. It is easily made and there is no need to bake it. Simply take about three-quarters of a pound of raisins, a pound of figs, a pound of dates, three-quarters of a pound of prunes, mix it all together, either by hand or with a food processor and roll into a small and round loaf of bread. Roll it in some freshly shredded coconut and slice as desired. It should be kept under refrigeration until used.

I also pointed out that eggs and raw milk are natural foods too. While the raw milk of goats is more nourishing than cow's milk, so long as the milk is raw and certified to be healthy milk, it is much superior to processed milk.

For eggnog, take a cup of raw cold milk, one raw egg and a teaspoonful of vanilla and combine in a blender. After blending for a few seconds, add a little honey and some carob powder and blend a little more. The result is a delicious and nutritious drink that is easy to digest and provides ample quantities of vitamins and minerals. Unfortunately, the fat content is high, so overweight individuals should use skimmed milk rather than whole milk. It will taste just as good.

And what is more delightful for dessert than a banana-strawberry pie? Who ever said that natural-food eaters can't enjoy living? First, make a crust out of some freshly shredded coconut, some ground almonds and finely chopped dates, all mixed together and pressed into a pie plate. Let it stay in the refrigerator to harden for about 30 minutes. In the meantime, get the filling ready. Take a box of strawberries, clean and slice them and combine with a little honey. Chop up a banana or two and mix with the strawberries and pour into the crust. You may or may not want to add some yogurt over the top of the mixture to make the delightful even more delicious.

As for luncheons and dinners, I told Patricia that there was no limit except her imagination. "For ideas, there are many good cookbooks with recipes for natural foods," I told her.

As an example, I told Patricia how to make a delicious prune salad, with walnut meats, bananas, melon balls and honey in a cradle of lettuce.

First, get some large prunes and soak them in either distilled water or bottled water. Never use tap water for drinking or for food preparation. Too often the cities add too many chemicals to the water. Cut the prunes with a sharp knife and remove the pits. Fill the prunes with chopped walnuts or other nuts. Cut a banana or two (depending upon how many people are to be served) into tiny pieces. Take the filled prunes and cut them into halves, then cut them into halves again. Cut up a cantaloupe or other melon into small balls and mix it all together. Pour some honey over the mixture, place over some lettuce and serve.

I also told Patricia how to prepare some other good and tasty natural recipes. For example, to cut down on appetite and at the same time to ingest some wonderfully nutritious food, there is the yeast cocktail. Brewer's yeast is literally loaded with all kinds of nutrition-rich food value such as inositol, needed to control body fat; niacin, needed by the body to convert sugars and starches into energy; PABA (para-aminobenzoic acid), needed by the thyroid gland and known as H_3, the youth-restoring vitamin; thiamine, an aid to niacin in converting carbohydrates into energy; pyridoxine, needed for muscular tone and for proper functioning of the pancreas; cobalamin, also known as vitamin B-12, needed in the body for production of red blood cells and to prevent general malnutrition; biotin, a powerful cellular stimulant; and pantothenic acid, also known as calcium pantothenate, a deficiency of this vitamin often causing constipation and various other digestive orders.

The yeast cocktail is prepared by combining equal portions of brewer's yeast with dry, skimmed milk and some water or fruit juice. The mixture can be stirred with a spoon until all of the dried substances have been blended with the water or some fruit juice. The resulting product will mix better and easier if a blender is used. The cocktail is a fine opener before dinner; it curbs the appetite because of its satisfying of bodily requirements. As you enjoy the balance of the dinner, you can do so leisurely and chew the food thoroughly and swallow slowly, mixing well with congenial conversation. Too often, people on a diet will gulp food quickly because of a strong desire to satisfy what they consider to be pangs of hunger. The cocktail or any other drinks should be sipped slowly so as to allow the salivary juices to mix with the food elements.

I urged Patricia to experiment with all varieties of fruits, vegetables, nuts and seeds. (Grains are included within the seed category.) Another nutritious cocktail, using pineapple juice, preferably juice from fresh pineapples, is made by pouring a cup of pineapple juice into the blender, adding three cabbage leaves, one-half of a fairly larged sized carrot, one celery stalk, one-half of a banana, one-half of a lemon (peeled), one-half of a fresh beet and one teaspoon of whole wheat flour. Run the blender until the mixture is well-liquefied. Some powdered milk may be added for additional flavoring and richness.

The nutritive and yet nonfattening qualities of such a mixture are astounding. Pineapple juice is rich in potassium, calcium and sodium. The sulfur and chlorine content makes it a valuable cleanser. The citric, malic and tartaric acids in the juice aids digestion and has a diuretic action, tending to remove water fluids from the body. Crushed pineapple also makes a fine dressing for salads.

Because of the high sulfur and chlorine content, cabbage is a good cleanser of the intestinal tract. Although cabbage is said to produce gas in the intestines and lower bowels, it is believed that this occurs due to insufficient mastication and the presence of waste matter in the digestive tract, according to Dr. N.W. Walker, a nationally famous nutritionist. Cabbage also contains calcium, potassium, iron and silicon.

The carrot is one of the most valuable foods, containing all of the elements and vitamins needed by the body. It is said to be an excellent cleanser of the liver. Dr. Walker recommends at least a pint of carrot juice daily. This juice also contains calcium, sodium, potassium, iron, magnesium, manganese and phosphorus, the latter said to be an excellent brain food. In addition to protein and carbohydrates, carrots contain vitamins A, B, C, D and G. (Vitamin G is also known as riboflavin and is often referred to as vitamin B-2).

Both the celery stalk as well as the green celery leaves are valuable. The leaves contain a valuable ingredient of insulin and the stalk contains organic sodium chloride (salt), which is far superior to ordinary table salt, an inorganic substance. Celery juice is an especially good drink in hot weather when perspiration causes a considerable loss of body salt. Celery contains vitamins B, C and G as well as some protein, carbohydrates, calcium, iron, phosphorus and potassium.

The half a banana in the cocktail is a fine energy source, much better than candy, cola or coffee. In addition to vitamins A, B and C, the banana contains protein, carbohydrates, calcium, iron, phosphorus and potassium. Bananas should be eaten only after spots appear on the skin, indicating ripeness.

The lemon juice in the cocktail provides a strong alkaline effect on the digestive system, despite the common impression that lemon, because of the citric acid contained in it, is an acid fruit. Lemon juice is considered to be very helpful for weight reduction, assisting the body in the digestive processes and preventing accumulation of fatty deposits.

One half of a beet in the cocktail adds blood-building nutrients to the mixture and has been reported as excellent for the kidneys and bladder. The teaspoonful of whole wheat flour into the cocktail provides the vitamin E that everyone needs. An important function of this vitamin is to metabolize excess fats and it is therefore of great value to anyone seeking to reduce weight.

Adding a tablespoonful or two of powdered milk (skimmed milk variety is preferred, for the smaller fat content), adds protein, carbohydrates, calcium, lime, phosphorus, magnesium, potassium, sodium, chlorine and iron.

Patricia made numerous notes during our various discussions about a diet of uncooked foods. She visited health food stores and was able to locate numerous health books with recipes for preparing foods without heating the food.

"But is it all right to eat cold food?" Patricia asked. "Does it not make it difficult for the body to have to digest cold food?"

I pointed out to her that the food attains body temperature by the time it reaches the stomach. First of all, the food is not simply poured directly into the stomach. It is taken into the mouth, a bite at a time, and if properly masticated and chewed until it reaches a watery state, the food is pretty well brought up to body temperature by the time it is swallowed.

"Do you mean to say that I am supposed to chew my food until it becomes watery?" she asked.

"One of the greatest mistakes that people make," I replied, "is the failure to chew food thoroughly. Thorough chewing or mastication enables the salivary juices in the mouth to mix well with the food and allows it to be properly prepared for additional processing in the second stage of digestion, which takes place in the stomach."

Not surprisingly, Patricia gradually reduced her weight with her new diet. She got rid of that superfluous 35 pounds she had been carrying around with her, which had been placing a strain on her heart and clogging her tissues, organs and blood vessels with dangerous fatty deposits.

In adopting her program of ingestion of uncooked foods, Patricia added herbs and spices to her food to improve the taste and flavoring of the food even more than before.

Patricia took up tennis and learned to combine recreational exercise with her choice of diet. By enjoying ideal health, she was able to carry on her duties as a wife, mother and executive secretary without difficulty.

HERBS IN DIETS THROUGHOUT THE WORLD

Some people may believe that the use of herbs and spices is a recent innovation started by a few young people in southern California. Actually, the use of herbs is mentioned in the Bible in many places. In fact, America was discovered as a result of searching for a new route to India, famous for herbs and spices.

China is also well known for its use of native-grown herbs, especially ginseng, and countries throughout Europe have long used garlic, peppers, mint, thyme, chives, basil, dill, rosemary, parsley, sage and many other herbs and spices.

Herbs and spices may have different names in different countries but basically they are the same plants. Time and finances permitting, I would love to visit various parts of the world and then write about the herbs and spices that are grown and used.

Chapter Six

Suggestions
for Breakfasting

It is not so much what you eat as what you shouldn't eat.

Dr. Paul Bragg

UNLESS you are already a master nutritionist, it would be premature to tell you of the ideal breakfast and expect you to follow the regimen of ideal eating. It is just too difficult to do. Therefore, I will seek to wean you away from bad eating habits. I do this at the risk of censure from some of my associates in dietetics, who may raise their eyebrows at my permissiveness. But, after all, food being as expensive as it is, I will usually allow my patients and readers to exhaust their supplies of forbidden foods and to try to refrain from purchasing any more of them.

SOME BREAKFAST IDEAS FOR THE SLIMMING DIET

When you are truly ready for the slimming diet and have consumed or otherwise rid yourself of the fattening and toxic foods such as refined sugar or sugar products; white flour and white flour products; commercial dry cereals; oleo margarines; fresh pork and pork products; smoked fish or smoked ham; bacon or sausage; lunch meats such as hot dogs, salami,

105

baloney, corned beef or pastrami; or coffee, with or without caffeine, you can then start eating and drinking what you ought to eat and drink.

This does not mean that breakfast time will be time to dread, with unappetizing food hardly fit to swallow. On the contrary, breakfast on the slimming diet will make you welcome the start of each day as you awaken.

Breakfast can be wonderful! There is no law that says you must have certain so-called "breakfast foods" such as ham and eggs, cornflakes or buttered toast and coffee. The reason for ingestion of food, aside from the pleasure of eating and drinking, is to nourish and sustain the body. Unless you are on a carefully planned fast, which we will discuss later, you should give your body, each day, all of the protein, carbohydrates, fat, vitamins and minerals needed for optimum good health. A part of each of the needed nutrients should be furnished your body at each meal, so that at the end of the day the required nutrients have all been provided.

Start the day with some kind of fresh fruit. Make it a generous portion, so that you can get that satisfied feeling when breakfast is finished. Don't be the one who eats a slimming breakfast at home, then stops at the restaurant for the regular breakfast.

If you do not already have a blender, see about getting one right away, because you are going to need it. Look for food processors. These machines not only blend but also slice and shred foods. Very convenient!

You might try to make a meal of a pound of cherries, if they are in season and if you can get the dark ones, which have more magnesium, iron and silicon than the lightly colored cherries. Cherries are great for cleansing the blood system, stimulating the secretion of digestive juices and effectively cleaning the liver and kidneys. Cherries also contain vitamin A, the B vitamins, thiamine, riboflavin and niacin, vitamin C, protein, carbohydrates, calcium, iron and phosphorus. The cleansing action of cherries is considered to be especially valuable for anyone wishing to reduce.

Similarly, you can make a meal out of watermelon, cantaloupe or other melon. In addition to a wide variety of minerals and vitamins and beneficial health action, the taste of fresh fruit for breakfast is always welcome. There is no reason why some fruits cannot be cut and mixed together into a fruit salad, such as cantaloupes, cherries, watermelon, pears, apples and other fruits and berries.

If the coffee habit is strong enough that you must have some "coffee," try a good substitute. Take a teaspoonful of blackstrap molasses and pour into a cup of hot water. Stir and allow the mixture to steep for about a minute. If it is not strong enough to suit your taste, add another teaspoonful.

Another coffee substitute is roasted dandelion root, usually available at health food stores. Yellow soybeans may also be roasted and made into a coffee substitute. After roasting until the soybeans turn brown, they are allowed to cool and then ground into powder or placed into a blender and made into powder. About a tablespoonful of the powdered soybean makes a good coffee substitute.

If the desire for cereal is strong, make some oatmeal or whole wheat hot cereal. Sprinkle with some cinnamon instead of sugar. Add some honey, if you want to sweeten the cereal. If you need some liquid, use some fruit juice instead of milk, to avoid the fat in the milk. If you must have milk with your cereal, try to get used to powdered skimmed milk, making some milk as you need it and keeping the powder in your refrigerator to avoid spoilage.

As for eggs and buttered toast, it may be difficult to break from this habit if you have grown accustomed to these articles of food over the years. However, eggs have so many valuable minerals and vitamins that the harm of eating eggs is minimal. There has been a great deal of controversy about the cholesterol in eggs but recent studies have revealed that cholesterol is a necessary nutrient and is manufactured by the body when needed.

So far as butter and toast are concerned, butter is better than margarine for several reasons, provided that the butter is recently churned and no preservative has been added, such as salt, for a long shelf life. Margarine is customarily colored to resemble butter and there is uncertainty with regard to the possible danger of this additive. There is also some question with regard to other additives that may be added to margarine during the manufacturing process and the value, if any, of the actual margarine.

If a slice of toast is needed, be sure to get whole wheat bread. Read the label carefully to make sure that no preservatives or coloring has been added. Another point to look for is wording on the label to indicate that there is other flour in addition to whole wheat flour. In such a label, the bakery could legally use undesirable cheap flour to a large degree and only a small amount of the whole wheat flour.

Sprinkle the buttered toast with wheat germ for a rich supply of vitamin E and choline, one of the vitamin B complex considered highly important for proper digestion. In fact, wheat germ should be sprinkled on many foods, including cereals.

Some other suggestions for breakfast include slicing a banana and sprinkling shredded coconut over it, with a topping of yogurt; boiling some brown rice and adding some powdered milk to it, with a sprinkling of honey for taste; or a bowl of sprouts.

Sprouts make an ideal food for breakfast, lunch or dinner. In addition, for the dieter who is always hungry, sprouts are fine for snacking throughout the day. You can use sprouts from mung beans, alfalfa seeds, sunflower seeds, garbanzo beans, lentils, soybeans and fenugreek seeds.

Sprouts are most nourishing when they are about one inch long. They can be sprinkled with your favorite herbs or covered with yogurt.

My own favorite sprouting method is to place a paper towel on a plate and wet a section of it. The seeds or beans are then sprinkled over the towel, after which another section of paper towel is placed over the seeds. Water is then sprinkled over the top so that both sheets are well moistened. One of the four corners of the towel is placed so that it will dip into a small saucer of water. The other three corners are turned up and over toward the center of the dish so that water will not drain from the towel onto the table.

By using this original method of sprouting, there is no need to constantly drain and rinse the water and the seeds, and in two or three days the sprouts will be ready to eat. It will be necessary to add some water to the water dish about twice a day to replenish the water on the towels lost by evaporation, thus bringing fresh water to the sprouts.

THE DANGERS OF MUCUS-FORMING FOODS

In 1912, a German college professor, Arnold Ehret, fell ill. Unable to obtain help from medical doctors, he tried various diets of his own, based upon studies of natural therapies. Professor Ehret, after trying many diets, decided that fruit dieting and fasting was the ideal program for any dieter wishing to regain normal weight and normal health as well. For example, he believed that a meal of two pounds of cherries contains enough nourishment to sustain the body for several days without any other food. He recommended having a meal of figs before or after a fast of several days. A diet of grapes alone was also tried, with good results.

The views of Professor Ehret with regard to diet and fasting are of a rather extreme nature and are to be regarded with caution. Fasting is a subject unto itself and involves preparation for the fast, fasting with herbal teas and termination of the period of fasting rather slowly and with mild foods. It would probably require a separate volume to explain proper fasting.

Disregarding his views on fasting, Ehret's teachings can be summarized by stating that he considered fruits and vegetables to be free of mucus-forming elements and to contain all of the life-supporting ingredients needed by body tissue.

Professor Ehret came to the United States shortly before World War I to visit the Panama Exposition. When the war started he decided to remain in the United States. He was especially interested in the nutritive values of the fruits and vegetables grown in California.

He believed strongly in cooked or raw green leaf vegetables, raw and cooked fruits as the ideal diet. He taught that the ideal foods are raw fruits and vegetables. He called this the "mucusless diet." Professor Ehret acknowledged that there should be a transitional period or time of adjustment to the new way of eating and drinking.

Ehret taught that certain vegetables, when raw, combined well with fruits and that others did not combine well. Vegetables that may be eaten with fruits, according to Ehret, are celery, lettuce, carrots and beets. He urged the use of one fruit or vegetable as the main or prevailing food and not more than two other fruits or vegetables as part of the combination. Although combinations are permissible, Ehret taught that it is best to eat only one fruit or vegetable at a meal.

For an acid stomach, which he referred to as a "mucused" stomach, he recommended grated or shredded raw carrots as the prevailing food, with the option of celery or beets if carrots are not available, and very ripe bananas, some raisins or sliced dried figs as secondary foods in the combination.

Professor Ehret recommended for use as salad dressing olive oil or some other good salad oil mixed with lemon juice. He also recommended the use of finely sliced green onions for addition to salads and the use of homemade mayonnaise, using lemon instead of vinegar.

To make mayonnaise, he suggested beating one egg thoroughly for about five minutes and then adding very slowly a pint of good salad oil, followed by lemon juice, salt and pepper.

The writings of Professor Ehret do not reveal any discussion of herbs or spices, but some good herbs and spices for salads are sage, thyme, marjoram, dill and garlic powder.

HERBS AND SPICES IN BREAKFAST FOODS

To those wishing to start toward the ideal diet gradually, it is necessary to learn the names of the herbs and spices appropriate for use on all varieties of foods for breakfast.

For example, a delightful spice over bread and butter is cinnamon. Before the dangers of sugar became widely known, it was customary to mix some cinnamon with sugar and then sprinkle it over the bread and butter to produce a tasty combination. Now that refined white sugar has been exposed as a destroyer of body nutrients and must never be used under any circumstances, even during a transition diet, substitute some honey for the sugar. You may use brown sugar if you have some on hand but remember the rule of exhausting the supply of undesirable foods and avoiding the purchase of such foods.

Other breakfast herbs and spices include pepper, especially the red pepper, cayenne. Black pepper is also popular, as well as onion salt, garlic powder, chopped, fresh parsley and chopped chives.

Freshly ground herbs and spices lose very little of their flavors and taste. It is best to have a small hand grinder for freshly grinding whole peppercorns. Many restaurants provide their waiters and waitresses with small hand grinders for grinding black pepper directly onto foods such as salads. Small chili peppers, ranging from red to yellow in color, are ground into the cayenne pepper. White pepper is more mild, being ground from vine-ripened pepper berries, whereas black pepper is made from unripened red-colored berries of the pepper vine. These berries turn black after they are dried. The white pepper is white because the black hulls have been removed.

Chopped, shredded or powdered mint is often used on many breakfast dishes. Savory, an herb of the mint family, is often sprinkled on various foods.

If you like to make your own breakfast rolls or bread, you will probably want to buy some poppy seed. Spread them on your work table and roll the biscuit or bread dough over the seeds just prior to baking. Poppy seeds may also be sprinkled over various foods for the delightful taste they impart. Incidentally, there are no narcotics in the seed itself.

Any of the herbs and spices mentioned may be mixed with the usual breakfast cereals or egg dishes or sprinkled over some morning tomato juice.

Other spices that may be used are marjoram, oregano and thyme. For a sweet flavor, use celery seed, which has a mildly sweet flavor. The sweetness can be too intense if used in an excessive amount, so use it sparingly.

In addition to qualities of flavoring and fragrance that herbs and spices add to the food, there are numerous other benefits to the digestive system and the body generally. It would make this volume too lengthy to delve deeply into these benefits and my book, *Modern Encyclopedia of Herbs,* tells of these medicinal benefits.

It is impossible to divorce nutrition from health because good nutrition is vital to good health. Likewise, for a lasting interest in good nutrition, it is important to understand, at least superficially, the effects of herbs and spices when used with foods or in drinks.

HOW HELEN J. AVOIDS DIGESTIVE PROBLEMS BY AVOIDING MILK

Helen J. was confused. "I see all these ads about drinking a quart of milk a day and the way the ads read they seem to be recommendations of medical doctors. Yet, when I drink milk, it makes me feel bloated, days will go by without a bowel movement and I have little appetite. Is milk causing these problems?"

I explained to Helen some of the dangers of milk. "Milk is rich in lactose, a disaccharide which yields glucose and galactose. These are sugars and that is what gives milk the taste of sweetness. For anyone wishing to avoid diabetes, it must be remembered that sugar is sugar, whether it comes from sugar cane, sugar beets, fruits, milk or other sources."

I explained to her that boiled cow's milk can cause constipation and that fat is predominant. Unless taken slowly and in small amounts at a time, the milk is liable to ferment. An acid stomach will curdle the milk. Also, bacteria acts on the lactose in the milk and changes it to lactic acid, resulting in the milk having an acid reaction in the stomach.

Human milk has an alkaline reaction in a baby's digestive tract and the curd of this milk is easy to digest.

After my discussion with Helen, she decided to eliminate milk from her diet completely. Mother's milk was fine for her when she was a baby and cow's milk is great for the young calf, but milk for adults or even for children other than babies is an unnecessary health hazard.

I told Helen about a recent newspaper report of the closing of a dairy because of excessive levels of insecticides found in milk samples. In addition, reports of bomb testing in China, Russia and other countries have indicated the pollution of the atmosphere with radiation, and radio-active "fall-out" has been known to fall onto meadows where cows graze. Of course, the ingestion of polluted feed affects the quality of the milk produced by the cows.

I explained to Helen that she could obtain the calcium found in milk by eating more vegetables. The leaf vegetables are especially rich in calcium and calcium is also obtainable from cheese, eggs and nuts.

WHY FRIED FOODS ARE BAD FOR YOU

In preparing breakfast, eggs are fried, ham and bacon are fried and many people also enjoy frying pork sausage or other meats. When pancakes are prepared on the grill or fry-pan, this too is a form of frying and should be avoided. If waffles are baked in a waffle-iron and are not overbaked so as to have the appearance of "deep golden brown," waffles may not be unhealthy, especially if made with buckwheat or whole wheat flour. Incidentally, some herbs may be mixed into the waffle recipe, such as mint, cinnamon or cloves, to obtain a special flavor and aroma.

The intense heat of the grill or fry-pan converts the food and the oil used in frying into an inedible substance that is suspected of causing cancer when ingestion is attempted by the digestive system. It is of course logical to presume that nature never intended for the human body to seek to transform inedible or burned substances into valuable nutritive elements for the repair of damaged or worn-out cells or for providing energy for the muscular system.

The general rule to keep in mind is to place into the body only the food or drink that will be used for energy or the repair of body parts.

HOW MARGARET M.
HANDLES MEAL PLANNING

After several long discussions with Margaret M. about the importance of a well-rounded diet, Margaret conceived her own program for meal planning.

"You are always stressing," she said to me, "the importance of including in the daily diet all of the vitamins, minerals, carbohydrates, fat and protein needed by the body. Well, I've decided to take one-third of the daily requirements at each of my three daily meals. For example, I get vitamin A from my two eggs for breakfast. I may cut down on my egg portion and take only one egg and make up for it by taking more vitamin A during lunch or at dinner."

Margaret received vitamin B-1 or thiamine from the egg yolk and also from the whole wheat bread she had with her breakfast. A slight coating with butter gave her more vitamin A.

Vitamin B-2 (also known as riboflavin and vitamin G) is in the whole grain cereal Margaret had for breakfast every morning. This vitamin is also found in eggs. Grapefruit also has riboflavin in it.

Vitamin B-6, pyridoxine, is found in egg yolks as well as in whole grain breads. Therefore, her breakfast of grapefruit, whole grain cereal, one or two eggs with a slice of whole wheat bread, supplied vitamin A, thiamine, riboflavin and pyridoxine. Margaret would sprinkle a little cinnamon over the bread and butter and some mixed herbs over the eggs, such as mint, cayenne, cloves, garlic or any of a number of other herbs and spices. These made the food taste delicious.

She would also get vitamin B-12, known as cobalamin, from her morning eggs.

She would get vitamin C from grapefruit or, if she sprinkled red pepper on her eggs, more vitamin C from the pepper. For vitamin D, Margaret would try to get out in the sun for a while but if there was no sun out, she would get some vitamin D from the eggs. The eggs also provide vitamin E and vitamin F, the unsaturated fatty acid. Egg yolks also provide vitamin H, known as biotin.

Although vitamin K is found mainly in leafy vegetables, there is also some found in fats, oats, wheat and rye, foods often found in breakfast dishes as whole grain cereals. Vitamin P, citron, is found in vegetable juices as well as in lemons, when eaten whole.

Choline, another vitamin of the B family, is also found in egg yolks. The vitamin known as pantothenic acid is also found in egg yolk.

Of the minerals, Margaret would get calcium from the milk mixed with her breakfast cereal, fluorine from the yolk of eggs and also in milk, iron from egg yolk and the whole wheat bread, magnesium from milk and oatmeal, manganese from whole wheat bread, and sulfur from eggs.

We discussed her protein intake and we agreed that practically all foods have some protein value.

We also agreed that her breakfast foods did not contain all of the minerals and vitamins. For example, chlorine is needed to keep the joints supple and also prevents excessive accumulations of fat. It is found in cheese, celery, cabbage, tomatoes, endive, spinach, fish, alfalfa and sea vegetation, such as kelp. By making certain that lunch or dinner contained one or more of these foods, she would be able to get the chlorine she needed.

Copper is usually not found among the breakfast foods so Margaret would need to add to her luncheon or dinner menu some of the vegetables, such as potato, parsnip, carrots and many other vegetables and meats.

THE LIGHT BREAKFAST PROGRAM OF RUTH T.

Ruth T. may have stumbled upon the perfect breakfast!

She had learned well the principles of nutrition and had reduced down to an ideal weight. Best of all, her knowledge of nutrition enabled her to maintain the weight she had sought.

She phoned and asked me, "What do you think of my latest idea?"

"Tell me about it."

"Well, we know that a raw egg has many vitamins and minerals. Collard leaves are loaded with vitamins B-1 and B-2, riboflavin, niacin, vitamin C, calcium, phosphorus, iron, potassium, protein, carbohydrates and a small amount of easily digestible fat. Why not put the egg in a blender, add one or two collard leaves, a tablespoonful of brewer's yeast, a cup of unsweetened pineapple juice and a handful of alfalfa sprouts? Won't you then have a breakfast that will be a fine starter for the day?"

I pondered for a moment when she asked the question. Yes, this could very well be an ideal way to start the day. If collard leaves were not available, beet leaves would probably do as well or some other substitutes such as lettuce or celery. Comfrey leaves would be fine, too, for those who are growing comfrey in their gardens. Alfalfa sprouts are full of life and contain lots of protein, vitamins and minerals, too.

"You have a great idea, Ruth," I said. I told her of my thoughts about making substitutions, both for convenience and for variety.

The encouragement I gave her generated more enthusiasm and more ideas. "What about some other good combinations for lunch and dinner? Why bother with using plates? Why not just use cups? Use the blender to prepare all your food, and throw in the foods you need to get all the vitamins and minerals and enough protein and carbohydrates."

I told Ruth that many people do live that way but that for the vast majority it is quite difficult to break lifetime habits of eating with plates, knives and forks and one course at a time.

"But go ahead and try it," I encouraged. "See how you like it and tell me what it does for you."

Ruth did try it and later reported to me that it was working out fine. She used the blender for breakfast, lunch and dinner. She would throw in a tomato, sliced cucumber, cut-up bell pepper or whatever she had on hand. I encouraged her to use wheat germ for vitamin E and yogurt, which has practically all vitamins and minerals in it. I warned her that when food is concentrated, it is more important than ever to take a little at a time and swirl it well around the mouth so as to absorb the juices from the salivary glands. Also, by swallowing a little at a time, stomach juices have a chance to cope with digestion of the food as it enters the stomach from the esophagus.

At my suggestion, she seasoned her food-drinks well with all kinds of herbs and spices. This not only added to the flavor and fragrance but, as pointed out in my book *Modern Encyclopedia of Herbs,* many of the herbs and spices have important medicinal values that not only help to restore good health but help to maintain good health.

Chapter Seven

A Lunch That
Helps You Stay Slim

Investigators point out that if fat children tend to have fat parents, family eating habits could be involved.

Lawrence Galton

WHAT you eat for lunch could well be the key to health or disease. If you are going to eat foods difficult to digest and lacking in nutritional elements rather than foods that digest easily and are rich in elements that satisfy bodily requirements, you will probably get through the day but the stress and strain on your body's glands and organs will gradually break them down.

If you are careful in the selection of food and drink for lunch, it is very likely that you will also be careful in your selections for breakfast and dinner.

With a healthy body, you will be better equipped to carry on with your daily projects and to overcome the many daily problems.

VARIETIES OF SPROUT SANDWICHES

Have you ever heard of a sprout sandwich? Neither have I, but it's a great idea for lunch. Why? Because sprouts are rich in protein, vitamins and minerals, that's why!

Sprouts are whole foods because they are freshly emerged from seeds and seeds contain all the elements that a plant or the human body needs.

Fish has been hailed as a brain food because of its high phosphorus content. Well, sprouts contain about 20 times as much phosphorus as fish. If it is mental power you want, sprouts are for you!

Vitamin E is now widely recognized as a heart, nerve and reproduction vitamin. Vitamin E as found in sprouts is in its most pure and most effective form. If you are interested in regeneration, rejuvenation and recuperation, sprouts are for you!

The complex of the various B vitamins are important for the human nervous system, the digestive system and for healthy skin. Sprouts are rich in B vitamins. If you want a healthy body, sprouts are for you!

Salt is often taken away, on medical advice, from persons having heart problems. Sprouts are low in salt content. If you are concerned about the danger of salt in foods, sprouts are for you!

Which of the seeds should be used for sprouting? All of them are good but my favorite is alfalfa. Researchers claim that alfalfa has ten times more mineral value than any other grain. It is abundant in phosphorus, chlorine, silicon, aluminum, calcium, magnesium, sulfur, potassium and a small quantity of sodium, all in correct proportions and balance to build strong bones, sound teeth, healthy brains and an all-around excellent body.

You may use any kind of bread you wish for your sprout sandwich but avoid the white flour breads, which are often a cause of constipation. Rye bread is a favorite with me as it is a muscle builder and is rich in vitamin E, phosphorus, magnesium and silicon.

Sprinkle the sprouts with some appetizing spices, for a flavor and fragrance that makes eating so pleasurable. Try one or two herbs or spices at a time or try various combinations. Some more popular herbs and spices are allspice, asafetida, celery seeds, chives, cinnamon, cloves, garden burnet, garlic, ginger, mace, nutmeg, oregano, paprika, tarragon and thyme.

For the preparation of sprouts from seed, I have already described my own original method in previous pages. In addition, there are a number of manufacturers of sprouting equipment. A simple, home-made sprouting device is to place about a teaspoonful of alfalfa seeds (larger quantities for larger seeds) into a wide-mouth jar, add water to it and then cover with a cheese-cloth covering bound with rubber bands or string. Twice a day, pour water into the jar and pour it out again, the cheese-cloth retaining the seeds. It usually takes three or four days for the sprouts to emerge from the seeds. Most sprouts are ready to eat when they are about one-half inch in length.

ELOISE W. AND HER HERBAL LUNCHES

Eloise W. grew tomatoes and comfrey in her garden. Anyone not familiar with comfrey should know that it is an ideal salad food although listed in the dictionaries and encyclopedia as an herb. It is a fine replacement for lettuce.

Using sliced tomatoes, comfrey leaves and toasted rye bread coated with avocado, Eloise was able to produce a lunch that contained practically all the vitamins and minerals that she needed for good care of her body.

A seaweed known as kelp is a valuable herb after it is removed from the ocean, chopped and dried. It is usually available in powdered form and should be freely sprinkled on foods of all kinds. It is not only rich in iodine but also contains about 30 other minerals, including copper, manganese, phosphorus, silicon, vanadium, zirconium and many other elements needed by the body.

Eloise used kelp frequently on lunch foods and was able to maintain a proper weight and the good health that accompanies it.

There are thousands of valuable herbs suitable as food. Experiment with them and discover for yourself which are most appealing to you. Eloise has been trying out various herbs for over a year and is still trying out various herbs and spices on foods and beverages.

HERBS AND SPICES IN YOUR LUNCH BAG

The high cost of living has forced many men and women to seek employment, with baby sitters taking care of their children when they are not in school. Whether parents or not, the fact remains that there are numerous individuals who either have to pack a lunch or eat in public places.

Food in public restaurants is often expensive or of doubtful quality. It is hard to tell whether the vegetables in the soup are fresh or simply re-warmed from the previous day; whether vegetables served on a plate have been boiled so long that they have lost most of their nutrients; whether the hamburger being served is fresh meat or leftover.

To be safe and secure in the freshness of your food, pack your own lunch in a lunch pail or paper bag and take a supply of herbs and spices with you.

What should you place in the lunch pail or bag?

If you are overweight, you will want to eat lightly and yet obtain many of the vital minerals and vitamins that your body needs, as well as carbohydrates, protein and a little fat. At the same time, it is important to bear in mind the rules governing acid and alkaline balance.

One of the problems to overcome is the spoilage danger. You cannot take foods that will spoil unless there is a refrigerator where your lunch may be stored until you are ready to consume it. A small thermos jug will come in handy for a cold or hot beverage and there are some thermos containers on the market that will keep food from spoiling.

One solution is to prepare your food in a blender and to then pour it into a thermos jug to maintain its freshness. First, get some raw, live vegetables for your lunch and place some sprouts or one or two leaves of comfrey, lettuce or cabbage into the blender. Raw spinach is considered to be a highly nutritious food. It is extremely rich in vitamin A and also contains fairly high quantities of vitamin C and riboflavin (vitamin B-2). As to minerals, spinach is rich in potassium, sodium, iron, phosphorus and calcium. Lettuce and cabbage also have these minerals and vitamins but in smaller quantities. Comfrey is rich in calcium and many other nutritive qualities. In my book *Modern Encyclopedia of Herbs,* I explain how comfrey, because of the high protein content, has become recognized as a highly nutritious food. We need to recognize that herbs as well as spices are foods and have medicinal qualities.

If you are using a blender rather than a juicer (every family should have both) you will need some liquid before the leaves can be transformed into puréed form or liquefied. You may use one or two tomatoes for liquid instead of water. A large cucumber may also be used as a liquid base because of the high percentage of water in cucumbers.

Should you have the advantage of a juicer, you may want to make some carrot juice, extremely rich in vitamin A and containing many other vitamins and minerals.

Any number of herbs and spices may be used to flavor and add nutritive qualities to the drink, such as basil leaf flakes, celery seed, chervil leaves, clove powder, dill seed, marjoram, mustard seed, oregano leaves, chopped or flaked parsley, freshly ground black pepper, ground sage leaves, savory leaves, sesame seeds, tarragon leaves or thyme.

Try to prepare enough for one lunch and avoid storing the remains of the drink from one meal period to another. The longer fruits and vegetables remain uneaten, the more they deteriorate, even if kept in the refrigerator. Of course, if you want to keep a little juice in the refrigerator to sip between meals, that would be much better than drinking a cola drink, cold beer, soft drink or caffeine drinks with coffee or chocolate.

You can try all kinds of variations and combinations when preparing your liquid lunch. You might want to try celery for your liquid lunch. Combine parsley with the drink for oxygen metabolism and for improved hormonal functioning. Vegetable juice drinks are truly the fountain of youth.

HOW SAM L. LUNCHES AT THE DINER AND LOSES WEIGHT

Sam L. was really overweight. Sam was five feet, six inches tall and at that height, with a medium frame, he should not have been more than 143 pounds. His weight was 185 pounds, 42 pounds in excess weight.

Following my rule of first trying to convince this weight-loss client of the importance of eliminating certain so-called foods from the diet, Sam was slow in changing from lifetime bad eating and drinking habits but eventually the changes came.

Sam was a mechanic and the place where he worked had a diner on the premises, patronized by truck drivers and road travelers. Realizing that certain foods should be avoided, he was uncertain as to what to order.

"Finally," Sam told me, "I hit upon the solution. I would order a vegetable plate, with fresh lettuce and tomatoes forming a circle around the edge of the plate and with various cooked vegetables in the center of the plate, such as a baked potato, corn on the cob, zucchini, some bell pepper, cucumber slices, carrots and peas. Before long, the waitress would order for me without my having to tell her. Whatever vegetables they had on hand would be arranged for a full plate. I told them it was 'doctor's orders' that I eat this way."

"What about dessert?" I asked. "Do you ever indulge?"

"Only once a week—on Fridays, to celebrate the end of the week," he answered.

I did not protest his weekly dessert as I long have been lecturing on the need for a gradual change in lifestyle, based upon understanding and self-desire to change, rather than to have change imposed upon anyone. In time, as he learned more about the importance of dieting, he would himself stay away from desserts and other fatty foods with or without preservatives and dangerous food colorings.

As the weeks passed by, Sam's excess weight gradually disappeared. Of course, in addition to a vegetable plate lunch, spiced liberally with garlic powder, black pepper, red pepper, marjoram, oregano and several other spices, Sam was careful with his breakfast and dinner intake also.

USING SPECIAL SOUPS FOR SLIMMING

Nutritionists generally agree that a good soup is a meal in itself. A bowl of soup with a sandwich is too much food. Evaluate the food value of a bowl of soup and you will see for yourself that a good bowl of soup for lunch, or even dinner, is enough nourishment.

Take peas for example. A good pea soup contains practically all the minerals and many vitamins, except for vitamin C. A soup with lima beans also contains the vitamins and minerals contained in peas but also has vitamin C. In addition, both peas and lima beans contain vitamin B-17, known as laetrile, amygdalin and nitriloside, and there is a lot of evidence indicating that this vitamin is a factor in reducing the incidence of cancer.

Other favorite soup items are lentils, potatoes, tomatoes, carrots, turnips and cabbage. Spinach has been purposely omitted as an ingredient for soup. While it is excellent as a raw food, doing wonders for constipation sufferers, there is some controversy about its value in cooked form due to the presence of oxalic acid.

Favorite herbs and spices for soups include basil, bay leaves, burnet, caraway seeds, celery leaves and stalks, chervil, coriander, dill seeds and leaves, fennel, hyssop, leek, lovage, marigold, black and white peppercorns, summer and winter savory, sorrel and sweet cicely (which is widely used as a sugar substitute).

MURIEL'S HERB GARDEN
AND HER DAILY LUNCHES

Practically all herbs can be easily grown if you have a greenhouse. If you don't have a greenhouse, you may be able to grow herbs inside your residence in a box of earth near some window. The sunshine will bring its warmth and the magic of the sun's rays to the plant.

Of course, there is always the outdoor garden and that is what Muriel had. However, her growth season was limited to one planting. By the time the danger of frost was over and the plant started to grow and develop and the time for harvest arrived, it would be too late to start the process all over again. However, the grown plant could be cut, dried and preserved, and by using it sparingly, there would usually be enough for the next harvest.

Muriel planted in her backyard such herbs as lavender, rosemary, thyme, lemon balm, tansy, mint comfrey, onions and ginger. To repel insects, she planted garlic cloves in various areas throughout the garden. To protect tomato plants, she planted basil near them. Incidentally, basil has become well known as a fly repellent.

Muriel would start her lunch with an appetizing drink made with mint and lemon juice, prepared hot in the winter and cool in the summer. She would then take a tomato or two from her garden, add two or three comfrey leaves, some chopped onion and any other available herbs and place them in a blender. This resulted in an extremely appetizing and delicious drink that was full of natural nourishment. That would be her lunch.

After harvesting her herbs, Muriel had a simple procedure for drying them and putting them away for future use. She would simply pull them from the ground, roots and all, tie some twine about them into bunches and hang the bunches up to dry in the air. Sometimes, if the aroma was especially attractive, she would hang the bunches in the kitchen, imparting the fragrance of the herbs not only into the kitchen but throughout the house.

If some of the plants had heads going to seed and she wished to preserve the seeds, she would use some old paper shopping bags and then insert the seed heads into the bags, wrap some twine about the bag and the plant and hang the bag so that the bottom of the bag would catch the seeds as they dropped. She would allow the seeds to dry well before putting them away for planting again next year.

Sometimes, when in a hurry, Muriel would place some herb plants into the oven, leaving the door slightly ajar to allow the moisture to escape and set the oven a little over 100°F.

After the herbs dried, she would usually shred or powder them with the help of a blender. She would then keep them in glass jars, capped, to exclude oxygen. When she needed some herbs, there they were!

UNUSUAL HERBAL TREATS FOR LUNCH

Before discussing herbal treats, I should explain the meaning of the word "herbal." First, there is the narrow, botanical definition, found in the standard dictionaries; namely, that an herb is a seed-producing plant that grows annually, biennially or perennially. The woody tissue of the stem does not continue to grow but dies and decays at the end of a growing season.

Then, there is the broad definition of an herb as a plant useful to people for flavor, fragrance, medicinal, religious and decorative purposes. This is perhaps too broad a definition and a happy medium between the narrow and the broad definition must be sought. This book deals mainly with herbs as nutritional aids, not only for the flavor and fragrance they add to foods but also for the nutritional qualities, also referred to as culinary uses.

One fine treat for a spread over foods for lunch or even over breakfast and dinner dishes is a naturally made tomato ketchup. Place about a gallon of ripe tomatoes in a large pot. Add two whole peppers, one ounce of garlic, one pint of good vinegar, one tablespoonful of cayenne, two tablespoonfuls of allspice, eight tablespoonfuls of mustard seeds, four tablespoonfuls of cloves, one tablespoonful of mace and four tablespoonfuls of sea salt. Boil until half or nearly half the mixture has boiled away. Strain and then pour the liquid into a jar or bottle and cover tightly. The ketchup will be a treat on almost any food.

Another herbal treat is to prepare baked potatoes by first cutting the potato in half and rubbing each half with herbs such as marjoram, thyme, chives, savory, dill or basil. Inserting a slice of onion between the halves gives extra flavor. Put the halves together, wrap in baking foil and bake.

A highly nutritious seaweed and therefore to be considered is agar-agar, also known as Japanese gelatin, a seaweed normally found in Oriental waters. The ordinary gelatin sold in stores usually contains sugar and is therefore forbidden for use by lovers of natural foods. One ounce of agar-agar to 20 ounces of hot water constitutes a nourishing food for invalids as well as for healthy individuals. Add to it, before refrigerating, some seasonal fruits, cut into small pieces, and you will have a delicious treat in your refrigerator that will be free from any dangerous colorings, preservatives or other deleterious substances.

If you are expecting company and want to really impress them with an herbal treat reminiscent of old-fashioned gourmet delicacies, try preparing some hors d'oeuvres made with zucchini. Without peeling, slice the zucchini and lay on a baking dish. Sprinkle lightly with paprika. Take about four tablespoonfuls of peanut butter, mix with a mashed clove of garlic and a teaspoonful of minced or chopped parsley and a well-chopped shallot. Spread the mixture over each slice of zucchini and bake at 500° for about seven minutes. Your guests will be amazed at the delightful flavor and taste of this healthy treat.

A cold drink made with fresh mint blended with lemon juice and some honey will make a fine beverage for hot days that goes well with the hors d'oeuvres or without anything else. The same drink, heated, is great for warming up the body on those cold winter nights just before retiring.

HOW JIM W. RETAINS
HIS YOUTHFUL APPEARANCE

Have you ever met anyone who looked much younger than his or her actual age? Well, Jim W. was just such a person. He was 50 but didn't look a day over 40. How did he do it?

Jim told me the answer. "Dr. Kadans," he said, "I have spoken with you many times and listened to your public lectures. You have convinced me that the body must have all of the minerals and vitamins daily, as well as proteins and carbohydrates. I make sure that I get all of these things into my system every day."

He continued his explanation. "First, I had the weight problem. You convinced me that I was eating and drinking much more than my body needed. In the past, I would go on a diet, trying one and then another, but nothing seemed to work. Oh, yes! I would lose weight for a while, but soon it would all come back again and usually I would end up weighing more than when I started the diet. It was only after you educated me, little by little, that I finally realized I must eat and drink only what is good for my body and not what I enjoy eating. The most surprising part of the whole program is that the food on your diet weight-loss program is the most delicious food of all. You couldn't drag me away from this program."

It's the same old story. A person convinced against his will is of the same opinion still. Education is the answer. A man must be told why a rule must be adopted, not simply told to adopt a rule without an adequate explanation.

JUNE J. AVOIDS PROCESSED FOODS IN HER DAILY LUNCHES

It took a little while to explain to June J. just what was wrong with processed foods. She was surprised to learn that they included lunch meats and cheeses. In the past, June used to have some kind of lunch meat one day and the next day some kind of cheese.

I explained to June that in the processing of meats or cheeses, various chemicals are added to preserve the food and prevent spoilage. For example, the process of curing and smoking hams is suspect. Years ago, it was customary for a ham to be cured in salts, sugars and spices. The natural juice of the ham would form a brine or pickle. An alternative process involved soaking hams in a brine solution for several months, curing and smoking it for flavor and then drying it to prevent spoilage. Later, it was found that processing could be expedited by injecting solutions into the artery of the ham and then into the smaller blood vessels and tissues throughout the ham. Phosphates were added to the brine to allow the tissues to absorb more water.

A recent exposé of one supermarket's sales revealed that when hams could not be sold because they became moldy and putrid, the store manager would order them washed with "liquid smoke" to disguise the smell and the condition of the hams. They were then sold to the public, to restaurants and to homes for the aged.

An example of processing that has an adverse effect on food is the pasteurization of milk. Pasteurization of milk destroys more vitamin C annually than is contained in the entire annual citrus crop. Vitamin C deficiency can be overcome by such foods as raw onions, cabbage or other leafy vegetables. Unfortunately, these foods are not eaten often enough or in adequate quantities.

Perhaps the principal reason for avoiding processed foods, in addition to the use of questionable preservatives and food colorings, is the inadequacy of refrigeration. Some markets practice moving fish back and forth from the fresh fish counter to the frozen fish section. This could go on interminably, without end, and the consumer has no way of knowing what is going on, except when a former employee will write a book about the practices of the large markets, as Jon A. McClure did in his book *Meat Eaters Are Threatened*.

Ground meat, still popular with a vast section of the public, is often mixed with sodium sulphite, according to McClure. This gives the meat a bright color on the outside but it could be green inside. It is especially dangerous in hamburger because all of the meat looks good, inside and outside and the odor is destroyed by the sodium sulphite. This is recognized as a poison that can kill. Nothing helps the cause of the vegetarian more than the adulterating of food by the markets.

Chapter Eight

Suggestions for
Delicious, Slimming
Evening Meals

Nutrition is the sum total of all the processes and functions by which growth and development, maintenance and repair of the body and by which reproduction are accomplished.

Dr. Herbert M. Shelton

IT is truly exciting to learn that you can combine the rules of nutritive ingestion of food with menu planning ideas that produce delicious, nonfattening meals at the same time. One of the greatest obstacles to diet control has been the failure, in the past, to replace the sweet and fattening foods and drinks with delicious foods and drinks just as attractive, if not more so, as the prohibited items.

In most families, the main meal of the day is the evening meal. Therefore, this meal probably needs more attention by the meal-maker than any of the other meals of the day. This chapter gives you ideas for evening meals that should result in many compliments on your abilities as a cook.

In addition, the recipes are amply fortified with herbs and spices,

129

which not only lend flavor and good taste to foods and drinks but have the beneficial side effect of enhancing good health. This is not to say that only herbs and spices produce good health. All wholesome foods do that.

SPICING PLAIN VEGETABLES
WITH HERBS AND SPICES

It is important to know which herbs and spices go best with various vegetables. In the preparation of salads, for example, consisting of such vegetables as celery, lettuce, tomatoes, bell peppers, cucumbers, carrots and beets, the herbs most generally suitable for sprinkling over salads include chives, thyme, mint, tarragon, hyssop, oregano, cumin seeds, celery seeds, anise, summer savory, chervil, borage and garden burnet. The young, tender leaves of horseradish or fresh radish leaves, chopped or finely minced make the salad more delicious. Rubbing some garlic on the salad bowl, before adding the vegetables, enhances the fragrance of the salad feast. Every salad has a sprig or two of parsley to beautify and add flavor to the salad.

In selecting vegetables for salads, choose those that are most fresh and crisp. Much of the food value as well as taste is lost in vegetables that have wilted or shrunk. The vegetables should be well cleaned. Root vegetables such as carrots or beets should not be peeled or scraped but should be carefully scrubbed with a brush. The outer peelings have valuable minerals and vitamins that should be ingested.

Raw vegetables are abundant in vitamins and minerals. However, if they are shredded, diced, cut, hashed, sliced or otherwise broken, this permits oxygen to oxidize the vitamins, causing their loss and destruction. Oxidation is especially destructive to vitamin C.

While vegetable juices are not as wholesome as the whole vegetable, there are times when it may be desirable to drink the juice rather than to forego having any vegetables at all.

In preparing the salad, a variety of not more than three vegetables should be enough. Many vegetables have similar values with respect to vitamins and minerals and there is no useful purpose served in oversupplying the body. Dr. Herbert Shelton, a well-known nutritionist, is highly in favor of the "law of the minimum," a phrase used to encourage individuals to supply the body with elements of nutrition most urgently needed. However, with respect to the three vegetables selected, there should be ample amounts available to fully satisfy the appetite.

There are certain herbs and spices that go especially well with certain vegetables. For example, anise and clover flowers go well with beets. Many food experts also like to sprinkle mace on carrots, cauliflower, squash, Swiss chard, spinach and potatoes. Chives are generally chosen for adding flavor to cucumbers, lettuce and clover flowers, beets and is a favorite for sweet potatoes and tomatoes. Ginger goes well with carrots, onions and winter squash and sage is often sprinkled over tomatoes. Mint leaves, finely cut, are frequently spread over peas and potatoes.

When you boil potatoes, turnips, peas, or cauliflower, use fresh or dried rosemary leaves to flavor the vegetables. You may also want to tenderize, by boiling, such vegetables as onions, mushrooms, lima beans, string beans, corn, carrots, eggplant, pumpkin, varieties of squash, rice and spinach. Some of the herbs and spices commonly used in vegetable soups include allspice, anise, asafetida, basil, bay leaves, caraway, chervil, cumin seeds, dill, fennel seeds, garden burnet, garden marjoram, oregano, parsley, summer savory, tarragon, thyme, mustard greens, mint, borage, and rosemary.

For a dressing over a vegetable salad, oil and vinegar is most highly recommended. It is preferable to select an oil that is free of cholesterol, and there are various vinegars on the market suitable for mixing with the oil. Apple cidar vinegar is good as well as tarragon vinegar.

One favorite salad dressing is to use olive oil with apple cider vinegar, with about one cup of the oil to one-quarter cup of vinegar and with about two tablespoonfuls of chopped fresh mint added to the mixture.

Experimenting with salad dressings can be fun. You may want to try a combination such as a tablespoonful of freshly grated horseradish with two teaspoons of tarragon vinegar, about a cup of sour cream, a dash of paprika and, finally, a teaspoonful or two of chopped chives and a matching quantity of chopped parsley.

Another spicy salad dressing uses yogurt as the main ingredient. To a pint of yogurt, add about four teaspoonfuls of lemon juice, two tablespoonfuls of honey, one-half teaspoonful of onion juice and a dash of paprika. Stir well.

A basic French dressing is usually comprised of one cup of olive oil with one-quarter cup of red wine vinegar, to which is added a dash of paprika, white pepper, one-half teaspoonful of dry mustard and one clove of garlic. Stir vigorously and allow to stand at room temperature for about two hours, after which the garlic should be removed. In lieu of the garlic clove, a dash of garlic powder may be used, in which case it would not be necessary to allow for any absorption time for the garlic clove flavor.

The basic dressing may be used as indicated or condiments such as tomato ketchup, chili sauce or chutney may be added. The quantity of condiments should be from one to two tablespoonfuls, the amount to suit the taste.

Variations of the basic French dressing would be the use of various herbs added to the basic formula given. Some of the herbs suitable for use would be borage, garden burnet, capers, chervil, chives, fennel, parsley, scallion or watercress. One to two teaspoonfuls should suffice.

For those who prefer mayonnaise, despite the richness of this dressing, there is a combination of condiments and herbs that may be appealing. To a cup of mayonnaise, add three-quarter cup of chili sauce, a teaspoonful each of tarragon, chives, chervil and parsley, cut up finely, with a sprinkling of curry powder and paprika. All of the contents should be thoroughly mixed and then allowed to stand for several hours for the herbs to permeate.

A final word about salad dressings. While they do add flavor and fragrance to the meal, as well as vitamins and minerals, the vegetables can really be enjoyed for their individual flavors and fragrances. Salad dressings are not necessities but rather fall in the category of exotic or gourmet dining fare.

HOW ANNIE G. STUFFS HER GREEN PEPPERS

Although an ample salad provides enough nutrition to be a meal itself, anyone indulging in a lot of physical labor during the day's activities, such as the husband of Annie G., wants to have a little more food. This is especially the case when, after many years of heavy indulging in food, one's wife, after gradually becoming wise in food selection and preparation, changes from a policy of encouraging family members to eat all they can to a policy of eating the minimum amount of nutrients for maintenance of good health.

Annie learned from reading health books that it is better to be a little underweight than overweight. Her big problem was educating her family, especially her very busy husband who, as a construction foreman, often participated with his construction crew in heavy physical labor.

Annie knew that her husband would never be satisfied with merely a salad, so she went to the butcher shop and selected some lean pieces of meat for grinding at home. She did not want to take any chances on the possibility of the butcher shop grinder having some leftover fat in it from a previous grinding of meat, which would be given to her with her purchase.

Annie had purchased a pound of meat but she needed only one-half pound for a serving of three. First, she took one-half cup of brown rice, washed it thoroughly and boiled it for about 20 minutes in a cup of water on low heat. Usually, after all the water was absorbed by the rice, it would be tender enough to eat. If the rice absorbed the water and the rice was still not tender, she would add a little more water and allow the rice to cook a little longer.

Annie would preheat the oven, setting it at 350°F. She would then prepare the balance of the stuffing for her three medium-sized green peppers. To the brown rice, she would add one-half cup of tomato juice, four tablespoonfuls of olive oil, one-quarter cup of chopped parsley, one-half cup of chopped onion, one-half teaspoonful of paprika, one-half tea-spoonful of garlic powder or one clove of chopped garlic.

She would prepare the green peppers by slicing off the ends with the stem and then removing the seeds and ribs. She would save the seeds for spring planting in her garden. The ribs were chopped into small pieces and added to the stuffing mixture. The stuffing was mixed thoroughly and then stuffed into the peppers.

Annie would place the peppers into a glass baking dish and pour about one-half cup of tomato juice around the stuffed peppers. As the peppers baked, she would occasionally pour the liquid in the dish over the peppers. Annie liked to bake either white or sweet potatoes or yams with the peppers, all at the same time. She then served her husband, daughter and herself adding some freshly sliced tomatoes on the plate for additional coloring, flavoring and delightful eating.

FOOD COMBINATIONS THAT
ARE OUT OF THIS WORLD

Pleasing the palate is the pursuit of people all over the world. Now it is becoming generally known that the most delightful foods are foods that are close to the freshly ripe, naturally flavored state.

Not only is a diet with natural flavorings loaded with beneficial nutrients but it is the most desirable diet for anyone seeking to lose weight. When such a diet is also more delicious than the ordinary foods commonly used in the past, it is a diet that no one can afford to ignore.

In this chapter, I will confine myself to discussing evening meals and describe delicious and exotic dishes that are not only slimming but also so tasty that the most fastidious gourmet chef would have to admit that they are delightfully tasteful.

A remarkable aspect of tastefully prepared food is that the food is simple and easily prepared. Food can be nutritious without having to be dull. A small healthful salad of fresh vegetables, followed by a dish of hot vegetables, with perhaps a small portion of lean meat, poultry or fish and finally some mixed fruit compote and a herbal tea with lemon and honey constitutes an evening meal of unsurpassed nutritional value and taste.

Meals need not be expensive to be delicious and nourishing. If store lettuce is expensive, dandelion leaves growing in the yard or along the countryside make a healthful and tasty salad. Comfrey leaves, easily grown either in the garden or on the window sill, are a fine salad ingredient, highly nutritious and tasty.

Carrots, whole, sliced or grated, are often added to the salad for color, taste and health. To avoid the hardness of the raw carrot, carrots may be sliced into one-quarter inch thick slices, placed into a saucepan, with boiling water added to cover approximately one-fourth of the contents of the pan. Cover the pan and simmer for about ten minutes or until the carrots are tender. Remove the carrots and use them in the salad.

If you have one or two large cucumbers, peel them lightly to remove the skin. Too often, the markets will spray a wax over the cucumbers to preserve them and make them look well. Of course, if you grow your own cucumbers, eat the skin as well. The cucumbers should then be sliced lengthwise and then cut crosswise into small pieces and added to the salad.

Several other vegetables may be added to the salad such as finely diced zucchini, chopped scallions, thinly sliced or grated beets, sliced tomatoes or cherry tomatoes, green pepper, sliced or chopped, and some alfalfa, mung bean, chickpea or lentil sprouts.

There are an infinite number of other salad variations, just as there are numerous delightful salad dressings. One of my favorite dressings is made with an avocado and the juice of an orange or lemon. First, the pulp of the avocado is beaten to the consistency of whipped cream. The juice is then added slowly while the beating of the pulp continues. Pour over the salad.

Fresh yogurt is another salad dressing that may be poured over a salad. A light covering is usually preferred. To make the yogurt rather elegant, add some honey and lemon juice to it, whipping it all together. Sour cream may be substituted for the yogurt.

For hot vegetables to be placed on the plate with the meat, poultry or fish, you may consider potatoes, either white or sweet, yams, corn, asparagus, brown rice or cooked chickpeas. There are other vegetables that may be cooked or baked to place on the dish. While many vegetables are mentioned, usually only one or two of the vegetables are enough for a serving. Two are more commonly served.

Herbs to be sprinkled over the vegetables or over the salad include anise seeds, chervil, chives, garden burnet, hyssop, oregano, paprika, tarragon and thyme.

If, in addition to the fresh salad and hot vegetables, you would like some meat, poultry or fish, slivers of garlic and leaves of various herbs may be added to the food while being broiled or baked. No food should ever be fried because of the danger of ingesting food that has been exposed to the extreme heat of a frying pan or grill.

For a delicious dessert, a mixed fruit compote of pieces of pineapple, grapefruit, orange, banana, pear and strawberries, whatever is available, adds a natural sweetness to the dinner that is the epitome of epicurean delight.

Finally, a cup of herbal tea, flavored with a piece of lemon and a teaspoonful of honey, would be a fitting climax to a healthful and delicious repast. Some herbs suitable for tea include angelica, balm, sweet basil, bayberry, borage, burdock, camomile, comfrey, coriander, fenugreek, flaxseed, ginseng, golden seal, horehound, juniper berries, magnolia bark, marjoram, mullein, parsley, peppermint, red clover, rosemary, sage, sarsaparilla, sassafras, senna, spearmint, thyme and yarrow.

HOW MARTHA B. SERVED
DELICIOUS LOW-CALORIE DINNERS

Martha B. did not frequently enterain dinner guests but it did happen occasionally. Her friends were not all health conscious but Martha always persevered in serving low-calorie meals when she did prepare dinner.

"Most of the time, they don't know they're being fed healthy foods. I never fry any foods or use white bread or sugar but no one seems to notice."

I knew that she was on a low-calorie diet in an effort to reduce, and I was eager to know how she managed to maintain her low-calorie diet while entertaining her friends.

"Don't they ever ask for sugar, coffee, cola drinks or other things that you have stopped using?" I asked.

"Of course not," she replied. "You know as well as I do that the rules of etiquette require the guest to accept or decline what is offered. It is not polite for a guest to ask for something that is either not visible or not mentioned by the host or hostess."

"What if they do ask?" I queried.

"I just tell the guest that I'm sorry but we do not have it. Of course, I always offer an alternative. If someone asks for coffee, I ask if he or she would like a delicious mint tea, flavored with lemon and honey. If someone should be audacious enough to ask if I have ice cream, I'll say 'No, but I'll soon be serving some delightful fruit gelatin.' I don't serve jello, because of the sugar content. I use, instead, the plain gelatin on the market, to which I add bananas, raisins, strawberries or whatever fruit is in season."

"Your avoidance of junk food is greatly admired, but just what do you serve as a main dish?" I asked.

"One of my favorite dishes is meat loaf or veal loaf baked and stuffed into cabbage leaves, grape leaves, lettuce leaves or papaya leaves. These are edible coatings, which the guest can eat with the meat. Sometimes, I will use a coating that is inedible but which will protect the meat and leave it tender and delicious, such as banana skins, palm leaves or corn husks."

"I understand," I said, "that a meat dish gives a guest some good and valuable protein. What do you include in the meat loaf to make it appetizing?"

"First and foremost is the use of the onion. Depending upon the number of guests I will be having for dinner, I will chop the onions finely, add a tablespoonful or two of finely chopped parsley and about the same quantity of finely chopped dill leaves. I usually add some olive oil as well as some uncooked brown rice. Also, I add about one-half teaspoonful of thyme, some garlic powder and a few grains of cayenne pepper."

"How do you keep the leaves from opening and the food from spilling out all around the oven?" I questioned.

"I will either tie the packet with some string or place it in the oven or casserole seam side down," she answered.

"That sounds delicious, but how do you keep your guests from overeating? Do you allow second helpings?"

"No second helpings," Martha answered.

"You say your evening meals are low-calorie," I probed. "How many calories do you serve in a meal?"

"Let me detail it for you. First, I serve a salad with lettuce, tomato slices, green pepper and carrots. Three leaves of lettuce equals about 15 calories, one-half of a medium sized tomato equals about 20 calories, one-half of a green pepper would be 10 calories or less and a carrot would have about 20 calories. This makes a total of about 65 calories.

"I avoid the Roquefort cheese dressing," she continued, "because this salad dressing alone would have about 65 calories. A tablespoonful of mayonnaise dressing would also have at least 65 calories and oil and vinegar dressings are just as bad, if not worse. A tablespoonful of olive oil, for example, would amount to at least 125 calories."

"I see that you have been a good student," I said, praising her. "But what do you do to the salad to add to the flavor and taste?"

"I refer to the section of your book (*Modern Encyclopedia of Herbs*) dealing with spice and herb cookery. Depending on which spices and herbs I have on hand, I will sprinkle on the salad one or two of such herbs as anise seed, celery seeds, chervil, chives, cumin seeds, garden burnet, garlic powder, fresh tips of hyssop, oregano, paprika, tarragon vinegar, or thyme. These herbs are not free of calories but the calorie content is very small."

"That's just fine," I replied. "But how many calories do you have in your main dish?"

"The meat loaf has about 260 calories and a baked potato 90 calories with about 25 calories allowed for a serving of cooked carrots. That makes a total of about 380 calories. Again, to flavor the meat loaf and side dishes of vegetables, I use some spices and herbs such as asafetida, basil, cinnamon, garlic, ginger, nutmeg, paprika, rosemary, tarragon and thyme on the meat (good for any meat dishes) and chives, cloves, ginger, mace, nutmeg, oregano, paprika, spearmint leaves and summer savory on the side dishes of cooked vegetables."

"May I say that I am highly pleased with your knowledge of which spices and herbs should be used for salads, meats and cooked vegetables. If more people would know about these uses of herbs and spices, there would be less sickness and more happy people," I commented.

SOME UNUSUAL DISHES TO SERVE

We are limited only by our imaginations. In selecting foods, we should always try to pick items that combine a variety of vitamins and minerals, to help meet our daily quota and to avoid the problems associated with deficiencies.

A food that is rich with nutritive benefits and highly appetizing as well is calf's liver. One of the healthiest ways of preparing it is to skewer it either in an electric broiler or over a grill. Before starting the broiling, you may want to first place the liver in some boiling water, cover the pan or pot and simmer until the liver is almost tender.

When ready, cut the liver into one-inch cubes. Peel some onions, the number depending upon the number of persons to be served and cut the onion into one-inch pieces. Also, cut up a green pepper or two to the same one-inch size and then, alternately, place pieces of liver, onion and pepper onto the skewers.

Many of the herbs generally used to flavor meats may be sprinkled over the liver and vegetables, such as garlic powder, cayenne or nutmeg. These spices impart a tasty flavor to the food.

Of course, the meal should be preceded by a salad of fresh vegetables such as lettuce, comfrey leaves, dandelion leaves, green pepper, tomatoes, celery, parsley or a combination of two or three of these vegetables.

Another unusual dish is to bake a mixture of dried fruit, such as chopped apricots, pears and prunes in a casserole with some lean stewing beef that has been cut into small cubes. The ingredients should be mixed together and baked in a covered casserole for about one and one-half hours with two cups of water and the juice and rind of a large lemon or two small lemons.

The fruit mixture should not be added to the casserole until after the beef has stewed in the water for about a half hour. This allows the meat to get a good start before you add the fruit. Some cinnamon, ginger or nutmeg or all three spices may be added to the fruit stew combination while baking.

After the meat is tender and the dried fruit has expanded, serve the food over some boiled brown rice.

For poultry lovers, preheat the oven to 350° and place the chicken or turkey parts in a shallow baking dish. Sprinkle with chopped mushrooms and chopped parsley; also, if available, some zucchini squash, celery, carrots or potatoes, cut into small pieces and distributed throughout the dish over the poultry. Some sliced onions over the top and sprinkled with some paprika or cayenne pepper would really do wonders for the taste and flavor. Bake, uncovered, for about an hour. From one-half to a cup of water may be added to the dish, depending upon the quantity of food and the size of the dish.

You may want to try baking some albacore, sea bass, bonito, butter-fish, cod, croaker, haddock, halibut, red snapper, smelt, swordfish, tuna, whiting or other sea fish in a covered dish, after first preheating the oven to 350°. These sea fish are chosen rather than fresh water fish because of the many rivers and lakes that have been polluted by sewage and chemical wastes. However, if you are certain that the fresh water fish comes from clean waters, by all means go ahead and use them.

Place the fish steaks or fillets in an ovenproof dish, pour some lemon juice over the fish, sprinkle with nutmeg and some pepper or paprika and bake for about 20 or 25 minutes or until done. Then sprinkle with chopped parsley, chopped chives and more lemon juice and serve. You may want to have some side dishes of cooked carrots, asparagus, corn or a baked potato.

Prior to each main dish, whether fish, poultry or meat, there should be served a platter of some fresh vegetables, seasoned with the herbs and spices that have been previously mentioned as specially suited for fresh vegetables, such as chives, garlic powder, oregano, paprika, tarragon vinegar and thyme, to mention a few.

For vegetarians, the dish of fresh vegetables seasoned with spices and herbs may be the complete meal, with the exception that the quantities should be larger than for persons about to eat fish, meat or poultry. Of course, vegetarians need to keep careful count of what is eaten to make certain that all of the necessary nutrients needed by the body are ingested daily.

For other unusual or exotic dishes, you may feel free to refer to recipes in cookbooks, magazines and newspapers. However, in doing so, it will often be necessary to modify the recipes so as to exclude any frying of foods, whether grilling or deepfrying. The intense heat associated with frying actually burns the oil or other material between the pan and the food and creates toxic and indigestible substances harmful to the body.

Be especially wary of cookbook references to braising of meat, poultry or fish. This is the method wherein the food is wiped dry and placed in a pan with enough fat to cover the bottom of the pan. The meat or other food is then turned frequently on a pan that is so hot that the food will sizzle. This is the browning portion of the braising procedure. After browning, the food is placed in a pan with about one-quarter to one-half inch of liquid, which may be fat from the browning or water or a combination of both, simmering over a tightly covered container.

To repeat, the braising method is described for identification purposes only and is not recommended for use. Slow and steady cooking of food is preferred. Always remember that the more natural the food, the healthier it is for the body. Cooking is necessary only to make food tender enough to make it palatable.

Most cookbooks are geared to please persons who know little or nothing about nutrition and who are unaware of the need of the body for simple foods containing all of the needed nutrients. References to sugar should either be entirely ignored or honey substituted, if sweetness is vital to the preparation. References to flour should be replaced with whole wheat flour or rye flour. When a recipe calls for milk, use raw milk if available, or use nonfat milk or low-fat milk. White flour has had removed from it much of the beneficial nutrients and whole milk contains too much fat for anyone wishing to maintain a slim figure and optimum health. One of the disadvantages of pasteurized milk is that the calcium elements in the milk, one of the chief reasons for drinking milk, are coated with fat particles by the heat of pasteurization, making it more difficult for the calcium to be assimilated by the body. Also, raw milk has live enzymes while there is nothing alive in pasteurized milk.

HOW TRAVELING SALESMAN JACK T.
STAYS ON HIS DIET

Jack T. is a traveling salesman. His work requires him to do considerable traveling both in small towns and large cities, mostly by air and sometimes by bus. His desire to stay on a healthful, slimming diet is complicated by having to eat in restaurants, airplanes or quick-food sandwich shops.

We talked about the selection of food in restaurants.

"I have followed your advice," he told me. "I avoid fried foods or food prepared on the grill. If they do not show broiled food on the menu, I will ask if they can prepare it broiled, whether fish, poultry or meat. If they have nothing but fried foods, I might ask for fried chicken, then be careful to remove all of the skin or other parts of the chicken exposed to the pan."

"How do you handle the situation on airplanes?" I asked. "There, as you know, all the food is prepared ahead of time."

"As a general rule, in booking a flight, I tell the travel agent or ticket agent at the airport that I want the meal for diabetics. Most airlines do prepare food for travelers who are on a restricted diet of this type. The food prepared for diabetics is usually of a healthier variety."

"That's fine," I said. "But suppose that you're in a small town and the only restaurant in town is in a hamburger shop, where fried hamburgers are sold on white buns, with cola or coffee the only available drinks."

"In such a case," he replied, "I will avoid the place like the plague. Instead, I will look for a grocery and make a meal out of some fruit such as bananas, apples or oranges."

DELICIOUS, LOW-CALORIE AND SLIMMING BEVERAGES

Drinking with meals, between meals, before meals and after meals seems to be a favorite pastime with many individuals. There are experts who say to drink copiously so as to wash out the system. Other experts say not to drink at all, it being necessary only to chew food well, pointing to the often made assertion that a very large portion of food is water.

My own belief is that it all depends upon the individual needs of the person. This is not the place to enter into a discussion of diseased bodily conditions in need of special programs of food and drink. Rather, let's consider various healthy drinks and beverages recommended to individuals who want to avoid toxic substances as well as fattening foods and drinks.

When I speak in this volume of drinks, I do not include in that category alcoholic beverages, beer or wine. All such drinks contain alcohol, which is not only rich in calories but is also injurious to bodily glands and organs that need to process everything entering the stomach. The kidneys and the liver are typical of glandular organs that are often adversely affected by users of alcoholic drinks.

It is difficult for many to realize that although some drinks may taste delicious, one has to choose between robust good health with long life and passing moments of a tasteful drink. It is true that some drinks have a lasting effect, such as alcoholic beverages; however, the harm that results from imbibing harmful substances outweighs the feeling of temporary well-being.

I cannot place too much emphasis on the point that the stomach has but limited capacity and that aside from the problem of drinking substances that may be harmful, and the problem of working the glands and organs unnecessarily in the processing of drinks of little or no value, we are missing the opportunity to correct unhealthy conditions and to improve our health if we fail to drink the many healthy drinks that are available.

For example, the problem of reducing weight is often complicated by poor functioning of the thyroid gland. This gland is largely concerned with metabolism. Unless fat in the body is properly metabolized and converted into energy, it is instead stored in bulges near the hips and lodges in the arteries, gradually building arterial walls and causing arteriosclerosis. Such a glandular condition makes it difficult to lose weight and also creates heart problems.

Metabolism functioning of the thyroid gland is greatly improved, according to Carlson Wade, a well-known health researcher and author, by the use of a herbal tea prepared with equal portions of golden seal, bayberry and myrrh. A small amount is prepared at a time, perhaps a tablespoonful of each herb and then well mixed. Only one-half teaspoonful of the mixture is then placed in a cup and hot water poured over it. After steeping for a few minutes, it is ready to drink and a cup of this thyroid-stimulating herbal tea should be taken one hour before each meal and at bedtime.

Coffee is of course a forbidden drink because of the caffeine content and the effect of caffeine upon the nervous system, kidneys and perhaps other glands and organs of the body. Some good coffee substitutes are on the market, made of nutritious foods such as barley or dandelion root.

Contrary to popular opinion, milk is not a healthful drink, except perhaps raw milk of the goat. Because of the fat content, even of goat milk, it is usually forbidden to persons seeking to lose weight. The calcium contained in milk is readily available from green, leafy vegetables. Low-fat milk or nonfat milk, is of course, preferable to whole milk.

It may help to understand what happens to milk when it is swallowed. Upon entering the stomach, milk has a tendency to coagulate or curdle. The curds mix with and cover other foods in the stomach and thereby prevent enzymes and other pancreatic digestive juices in the pancreas, located near the stomach, from reaching the food particles and digesting them. The undigested food then starts to putrefy and ferment. This often accounts for foul-smelling feces, which, in a properly fed digestive system, should have no foul odor. If milk is used at all, it should be taken alone, without other food.

For good digestion, the digestive system contains certain digestive juices called enzymes. In time, especially when a person places a heavy drain on bodily enzymes by failing to consume raw plant foods containing enzymes, the bodily enzyme production decreases. This, in turn, weakens the body. Enzymes have the power to produce chemical changes in organic substances by catalytic action. It is the breaking down of food particles that makes it possible to extract from the food the vitamins, minerals, amino acids, carbohydrates, hormones and other vital needs of the body. In the process of pasteurizing milk, the heat of the pasteurizing process destroys whatever enzymes may be in the milk.

I could write a book on enzymes alone, describing each known enzyme and its effect upon food and the body. However, it should be enough to realize that live foods must have an important share in the body's daily supply of nutrients, if the body is to be healthy.

While fruits and vegetables are alive with enzymes, this is not the case with canned produce. Canned food is customarily heated in the canning process for the purpose of killing all bacteria. In the process, enzymes are also destroyed.

I once attended a lecture by Dr. Ernst Krebs, Jr., who stated that he believed that a scarcity of enzymes in the diet is an important contributing factor in causing cancer. Dr. Krebs, a chemist, and his father, a medical doctor, are the scientists who co-discovered vitamins B-15 and B-17.

If you have a juicer and can get some fresh apricots, oranges, pineapple and papaya, you can prepare an after-dinner drink that your digestive system will relish beyond anything else you can think of. In fact, this drink is so rich in enzymes that will help in digestion that I would recommend sipping this throughout dinner, making it truly a fine dinner drink. Such a drink is far superior to coffee, tea, milk, the cola drinks or any other beverage. Indeed, it may be taken throughout the day, from time to time, before, during or after other meals of the day, for revitalization of the body. A similar cocktail may be made of vegetable juices on alternate days or alternately during the day, so as to help preserve the acid-alkaline balance in the body. Fruits are generally acid while green vegetables are usually alkaline.

A good vegetable drink is the carrot-celery cocktail. First, make some carrot juice and some celery juice and combine them in equal portions. A cup or two of this cocktail after dinner provides many minerals and live enzymes for the body's needs. Of course, the drink may be sipped during dinner. Minerals are extremely important because without minerals the vitamins in food cannot be used and properly absorbed into the digestive system.

If you feel somewhat constipated, make a prune milkshake by combining a cup of low-fat milk or raw milk that has not been pasteurized with about six prunes that have been allowed to soak for several hours. Remove the pits, of course, and then mix in blender. Do not strain out the prune skins as they contain valuable mineral substances. You cannot reduce if you are constipated. Bowel movements should take place at least once a day and the use of prunes, or occasionally soaked figs, will do much to keep you regular.

Thus far, I have failed to mention the most commonly used drink and yet perhaps the most dangerous. I am referring to tap water from the city faucet. Unfortunately, city tap water has had so many chemicals added to it in the process of "purifying" that I make it a practice never to drink tap water without first distilling it. It is fine for a bath or for washing dishes or the family automobile but not for the digestive tract.

I do not mean to say that because of the danger in the use of ordinary tap water, it should be avoided. If you can get a distiller or otherwise obtain distilled water, use plenty of it. It will help to keep you from getting constipated and will often relieve cases of constipation. This word of caution about tap water is prompted by reports of overchlorinating of city water supplies as well as the use of fluoride in the water, a chemical considered by many to be dangerous to the body.

Some signs of insufficient water, in addition to constipation, are fatigue, loss of stamina, fever, vomiting, diarrhea and irritableness.

In deciding whether or not to start using distilled water, you may want to consider the leaching argument used by the anti-distilled-water people. They argue that distilled water will leach the minerals from the body and thereby deprive the body tissue of much-needed nutrients. Advocates of the use of distilled water claim that if any leaching occurs, which they doubt, only the inorganic minerals foreign to the body tissue would be leached away; the organic minerals, the only minerals truly valuable, would not be affected by the alleged leaching danger. There you have it! Now, the decision is yours. If my own view of the matter would help you, I am in favor of distilled water use. I have a small distiller and use it constantly.

Before leaving the subject of beverages, I want to say a word or two about warm drinks, which seem to comfort the spirit as well as the body. In addition, fruit beverages have the quality of building resistance against disease. There are unlimited combinations to try. Depending upon the number of persons to be served, pour a quantity of apple juice, pineapple juice, and orange juice into a saucepan. Add some cloves, cinnamon and crushed cardamom seeds and simmer for about 15 minutes. While the heating will destroy the live enzymes, there is still a goodly portion of minerals and other nutrients in the mixture to make it worthwhile. For convenience, canned juices may also be used provided they have not had sugar or preservatives added. Fruit juices usually contain such vitamins as C and B-6 and such minerals as potassium, iron, copper, chromium and traces of other nutrients needed in the diet.

Another warm or hot drink is to place a teaspoonful of some cereal beverage into a cup, together with a teaspoonful of molasses. Then pour some hot low-fat or skimmed milk over it and stir well. Sip this beverage after dinner or just before retiring and you will likely enjoy a very restful sleep. Molasses is a rich source of iron and the amino acid known as trytophan helps you to sleep.

Instead of fattening milk for the little tots, it may be well for mothers to consider the recommendation of Dr. Are Waerland, founder of the European Waerland System for natural health. He recommends a natural food formula substitute for mother's milk, prepared by grating a carrot, a potato, some celery and parsley and boiling these articles for four minutes, together with the herb known as dill, in a pint of water. The liquid is then strained and mixed with an equal amount of raw, certified milk. This drink, taken as the first and last meals of the day, has the identical health-producing and long-life qualities of mother's milk, according to Dr. Waerland. It is suitable for grown-ups as well as for children.

Incidentally, Dr. Waerland's teachings provide for not drinking with meals because liquids dilute the enzymes and make them weak.

BETTY R. AND HER MEATLESS MEALS

"I'm so happy," Betty R. told me one day. "I never thought I would be able to get along without eating meat but I've managed to do it for six weeks and it's no problem at all. I've gathered together, from friends and cookbooks, a collection of meatless recipes and I feel fine. In fact, I feel better than I've ever felt before."

Betty had been grossly overweight and after several talks with her, explaining the dangers of being overweight, she became convinced and followed my advice. From a weight of 185, she reduced to 140 within a period of three months. Best of all, she was able to keep her weight down because she understood how the body functioned. By attending my public lectures and as a result of a series of consultations with her, she learned the science of nutrition and the need for supplying the body with daily nutrients and avoiding the overtaxing of the body with fatty foods, coffee, fried foods, sugar, alcoholic drinks, white bread, candies, cakes, colas and other junk foods.

"What is your best meatless meal?" I asked.

"There are so many good kinds of good meals, it's hard to pick one out. You've taught me that every well-balanced meal must contain some form of salad. Therefore, I always start both lunch and dinner with a vegetable or two, using lettuce, watercress, spinach, beet tops, radish tops, dandelion leaves, endives, turnip tops, mustard tops, kale, cabbage or parsley.

"Of course, I often use tomatoes. The tomato, as you know, has a valuable acid that serves as a solvent and aids in the digestion of other foods. Oregano is great for sprinkling over sliced ripe tomatoes. Powdered sage is also fine for tomatoes. For other vegetables, I like to use thyme and tarragon vinegar. Another dressing I often use on salads is a mixture of olive oil and fresh lemon juice.

"I said that I use only a vegetable or two, but that is a minimum. If vegetables are in season and the price is right, I'll have perhaps three or four or even more vegetables on the salad plate. Green plants are not only nutritious but they are highly ornamental as well. Salads promote digestion, purify the blood and help the body to grow healthy bones and tissue."

I was eager to learn how much actual cooking Betty did. I had warned her that cooking destroys enzymes and heating of foods should be kept to a minimum.

"Don't you ever cook any vegetables?" I asked.

"Of course I do! Who ever heard of eating raw potatoes or raw turnips or parsnips? Even asparagus has to be cooked. And of course, there are peas, beans, beets and sometimes carrots, although I prefer eating raw carrots, especially when they are grated and mixed with raisins."

"How much do you cook them?"

"As little as possible. Actually, just enough to make them tender and edible. This prevents destruction of the excellent nutritive qualities of the vegetables."

That was what I wanted to hear. I have often lectured on the dangers of overcooking. Too often, the best part of food is boiled away or poured down the drain during the straining process with the water remaining in the pot. I have often taken that water, poured it into a glass and saved it for later use as a nourishing and refreshing drink

"I didn't hear you mention corn," I said

"How could I forget? Corn has the purest carbohydrate in its most soluble form and has enough cellulose to encourage healthy movement of food through the intestinal tract. My favorite way of preparing corn is like making a soft-boiled three- or four-minute egg. First, I will get the hot water boiling and then drop in the corn on the cob for three or four minutes. That is all that is needed to produce the chemical change in the corn to make it palatable and delicious."

"So far, so good," I said. "But you know the danger of fatty foods. Don't tell me that you smear the corn on the cob with butter and salt, which most people do."

"Fresh sweet corn, prepared properly, without overcooking, is so delicious that it really doesn't need anything over it. Sometimes, though, when I have been good and have been watching my diet carefully, I might spread a thin coating of butter over the corn on the cob but, more often, I would simply sprinkle some herb mixture on the corn."

"You haven't mentioned cucumbers or onions."

"Well, just wait a minute. I can't think of everything! If the cucumber is store-bought, I will peel it to avoid the wax that so many stores spray on cucumbers. I love to make a cucumber and onion salad, slicing both the cucumber and onion and leaving them in cold water until ready to use. I will then place them on lettuce leaves, the greener the better, garnish with small radishes and serve."

"You don't use herbs over the cucumber and onion salad?"

"Of course I do! I use herbs on practically everything, not only to make the food tasty but also to add nutrients. I'm sure you know that many herbs contain all kinds of vitamins and minerals."

"Yes, I do," I replied. "But I'm just checking to see if you have been following through on the instructions I gave you."

Betty had been a good student and I was very pleased to note how well she was following the advice I gave her. I thought I would ask her about her aversion to eating meat.

"Betty," I asked, "why don't you ever serve meat with your meals?" The reason she gave was unusual.

"Did you ever see cattle slaughtered at the stockyards? They know they are about to be killed because they see what is happening to the other animals. As a result, they get excited, desperately seeking some escape. The adrenalin starts to pump through all of the tissue to give strength and courage to fight to preserve life. When sudden death comes, that adrenalin is still there, saturated throughout the body. And you know as well as I do that this is a toxic substance that can do nothing but hurt the body.

"Besides," she added. "I don't believe in taking life, even animal life. Furthermore, the tissue of every animal, man or beast, has uric acid and toxic poisons in the tissue that is in the process of elimination at the time of death. That acid and poison is taken into the body of the person eating that dead animal," Betty declared.

"Well," I replied, "I'll not argue with you. What you say makes good sense, although the great majority of people eat beef, lamb, veal, pork and poultry and many of them live long, full and happy lives. They also eat white bread, smoke tobacco, drink beer and other alcoholic drinks, drink cola drinks, eat candy, cake and products containing sugar, preservatives, coloring and other chemical additives of all kinds. I would like to see a statistical study made of the age of death of people who do these things as compared with those who do not. My guess, of course, is that the abstainers, like you and I, will live longer, will have more freedom from colds and other diseases and will better enjoy life."

HOW TO SELECT AND PREPARE MEATS

If you insist on eating animal flesh, there are rules to follow, just as the master of a vessel entering upon a voyage through dangerous seas should have navigation maps to guide him through the shallow and narrow places.

First, meat must never be fried. As mentioned before, studies indicate that the heat of the pan or grill becomes so intense that the meat surface contacting the metal is burned to the point where it becomes a toxic substance unfit to swallow.

Broiled meat, on the other hand, although subjected to considerable heat, is not exposed to the severe heat of the pan or grill. Furthermore, meat should be broiled only to the point where it is edible and not to the point where it looks a so-called "golden brown." When meat or any food, for that matter, is broiled to the point where it becomes dark, this signifies that the meat has passed the point of edibility and is starting to become inedible, the browning or darkening of the meat signifying an excess of heating and start of development of toxic substances.

Second, meat selected for the table should be lean. If it is packaged, remove the fat from the meat when you get to your kitchen. There will be plenty of fat in the tissue of the meat without any need for the visible fat around the meat.

Third, concentrate on organ meats such as the heart, liver, brains, kidneys and the pancreas (sweetbreads). The internal organs are richer in vitamins than the muscle tissue. Liver has a large quantity of vitamin A and also has a fair amount of the B complex and vitamin C. Meats generally are high in the B complex, especially in thiamine and niacin. The internal organs are also much richer in iron than ordinary cuts of meat.

Fourth, chopped meat or glandular meats should be used the day they are purchased or else frozen. Leftover cooked meat should be covered or otherwise protected from the air before storing and it should be used before there is even the slightest change in flavor.

Roasting usually applies to preparation of a large portion of meat such as roast beef or roast lamb. A large chicken or a turkey is also usually roasted. In broiling, the oven should be preheated for about five minutes and afterwards dried with a cloth. The meat should be be broiled from two to three inches below the heat, turning occasionally, with the door of the broiler slightly open. All sides of the meat should be flavored with some herb or two, such as thyme, basil, sage, chives or oregano. Many cooks like to also sprinkle with garlic or onion powder, or both. Sometimes, garlic cloves are inserted into the meat, using a knife to make small openings. Broil until tender.

For roasting, the oven is usually preheated to 325° and the meat allowed to roast at this moderately low temperature, allowing 10 minutes for each pound of meat. Of course, sprinkling with herbs, as in broiling, should also be done.

In preparing sweetbreads for broiling, it is best, after washing, to cover with boiling water and allow the meat to simmer in a covered pot for 15 minutes. The water is then drained, the pot filled with cold water and allowed to drain away again. The veins and membranes of the sweetbreads should then be removed and the meat again washed and drained. The meat is then dried with a cloth and placed into a preheated broiling oven. The sweetbreads may then be sprinkled with a salad oil, sprinkled with herbs and allowed to broil for about 10 minutes, turning occasionally. When served, a wedge of lemon is often placed on the plate so that some lemon juice may be squeezed upon the sweetbread.

In purchasing poultry, preference should be given to purchasing the white meat (breasts) as it is more easily digested than the dark meat, the fibers being held together less firmly. Also, the fat content is smaller.

In broiling chicken, wash thoroughly and dry one-half of the chicken (the broiler chicken usually weighs from two to two and one-half pounds) with a cloth. Preheat the broiler for about 10 minutes and then place the chicken into the oven and bake for the first 15 minutes at a high temperature of 500°, then reduce and bake until tender at a temperature of 375°. Sprinkle with herbs and turn several times during the broiling, which may take from 30 to 50 minutes.

USING THE STEAMER
FOR SOFTENING VEGETABLES

The problem often arises that there are vegetables at hand such as potatoes, turnips, parsnips, asparagus, beets, salsify, yams and sweet potatoes, all of the underground root and tuber family, but there is uncertainty as to the best way of tenderizing them so as to make them palatable.

One solution is a vegetable steamer. The food is placed into the steamer, with perhaps one-half cup of water. The advantage of this form of cooking is that there is no absorption of nutritive elements in the food into the water, which commonly occurs in the boiling of food.

Furthermore, there is no absorption of fat or toxic substances into the food, which occurs when frying. Fried potatoes, for example, may taste good because of the fat content.

It is so much better to prepare food without losing the health-giving qualities, which occurs in boiling, and without absorbing the fat-calories and toxic substances, which occur in frying. The liberal use of tasty and fragrant herbs and spices to food that has been steamed not only results in delicious and healthier eating, but the vitamins and minerals in the herbs are sorely needed by the body.

The use of the steamer need not be confined to tenderizing vegetables. The dictionary explains that cooking is a method of preparing food by heating it. It should therefore be apparent that in addition to vegetables other foods may be prepared in the same manner, such as fish, poultry and meat. The key to the method is the use of herbs and spices for flavoring and fragrance. These may be sprinkled on food while steaming or after removal from the pot, depending largely on whether or not you would like to have a delightful aroma of food and spices around the kitchen and dining room area.

Delicious desserts may also be prepared by the use of the steaming method. For example, instead of baking apples or other fruits, try steaming them. If you don't have a steamer, try to find some round rocks about one inch in diameter to place in the pot. These will enable you to fill the pan with water to a height of one inch and the food can then be placed on the cleaned rocks. The main point is to prevent the food from making direct contact with the bottom of the pot, thereby excessively heating the food and creating toxic substances. Be sure to cover the pot.

Food will usually be ready about the time the water steams away. I have tried this method of cooking with corn, yams, apples and other fruits and vegetables and it works just fine.

Remember, though, that it will taste better if flavored with herbs and spices during or after the food preparation.

EVELYN T. TRIES BREAD BAKING

By the smile on Evelyn T.'s face, I knew that she had good news for me. After a series of seven conferences with her, she had reduced her weight from 175 to 145 pounds. She still needed at least 10 pounds more to get rid of and that was the purpose of this conference—to discuss ways and means that she could reduce still further.

"Evelyn," I said. "You have a happy expression on your face. What has happened?"

"I did it!" she exclaimed. "I got rid of those surplus 10 pounds."

"How did you do it?"

"It was the bread. Remember, you kept warning me that the bread available in most all stores, even health food stores, is not 100 percent whole wheat flour or 100 percent rye flour and that if you read the labels carefully you will find that they do not claim 100 percent but that the label usually reads 'contains' whole wheat flour or 'made with whole wheat flour.' Well I've long suspected that these breads were not really as wholesome as I would like."

"If that is the case, then why did you keep on using the store-bought bread?" I asked.

"Two reasons," she answered. "First, I really enjoyed the taste of the bread. Second, I knew nothing about baking my own. Then I started reading books about bread making, especially those written for health food enthusiasts. And that's how I lost those 10 pounds!"

"You started baking your own bread," I said, rather assuredly.

"You bet I did, and it's easy. Anyone can do it. Not only do you get delicious, nourishing bread but it's at least half the cost!"

I was delighted to hear her talk that way. It had taken a long time. My pet theory in working with overweight persons is based upon the principle that the person must be convinced of the need for change in eating and drinking habits and that these changes must be brought about by a sound program of education.

"Okay, Evelyn. Out with it! What is your favorite bread recipe and explain it in a simple way because I may want to use in my next book."

"You ought to know the answer to that, Dr. Kadans," she replied. "After I read your book, *Modern Encyclopedia of Herbs*, Parker Publishing Company, Inc., I developed a bread recipe where you could use almost any of the herbs you name in your book and bring forth a most nutritious and wonderfully tasty bread."

I was highly pleased to hear her say that. I have long been teaching that herbs contain practically all of the minerals needed by the body, almost 100 in number. A few herbs mixed into the bread dough will not only make the food tastier and cost less to make but will have a highly nutritious effect upon the body generally.

"Just which herbs do you use and how much of each herb is used in your recipes?"

"I have a pantry full of herbs and usually use three or four with every recipe. Basically, the recipe is the same and it is only the herbs that I change. My favorite herbs are the onion, garlic, ginger, ginseng, cayenne, poke root, sarsaparilla, clover, licorice root, mullein, lobelia, hawthorn berries, carrot juice, carrot pulp and any number of other herb combinations."

"All right, Evelyn. Now we know about the herbs and spices you use. But what is the basic recipe?"

"It all depends upon how many loaves of bread that you want. If you are going to make one loaf, take one-half ounce of the wet (not dry) yeast and add it to one-half cup of warm water."

I wondered about the use of the fresh yeast rather than the dried yeast and asked her about it.

"Well, it really makes little difference," she replied. "There's a baker I go to that sells the wet yeast to me and I keep it in the freezer. It seems to last a long time and it's much less expensive. And I never seem to run out of it."

"Then for two loaves, you would double the quantity. Is that correct?" I asked.

"Yes, just double the quantity if you want two loaves and triple it if you want three and so forth.

"I let the yeast soak in the warm water for about five minutes. If you should decide to use the dry yeast, you could substitute a package of dry yeast for one-half ounce of the fresh yeast.

"After the yeast has soaked for five minutes, I add four tablespoons of a good vegetable oil or melted butter. Personally, I prefer the butter.

"I then throw in the herbs, usually limiting myself to two or three. If I use the onion, I would first grate enough onion to equal about one-half cup. I might then add about one-half cup of grated carrots and then about a teaspoonful of basil, thyme, chopped fresh parsley, nutmeg, cloves or any of the many other herbs that are so popular and tasty.

"After this mixture is all blended together, I stir in about two cups of whole wheat flour, using either an electric blender or a slotted spoon.

"I like to try different combinations of herbs in the bread, which makes bread making and especially bread eating an adventure in gourmet food preparation."

"It sounds easy enough," I said. "What do you do next?"

"First, I keep mixing until I have some dough. If necessary, I will add more flour until it feels like dough. I then spread a thin layer of flour on a bread board and move the dough from the mixing bowl onto the board. To keep my hands from sticking to the dough, I usually pour about a teaspoonful of salad oil over my hands and then move the dough ball round and round over the board and allow the dough to absorb the flour on the board, adding a little more flour now and then as needed. You will know your dough is ready when the stickiness is gone."

"What about all of the kneading that is usually associated with bread making, that takes so much time and really gives the bread maker a lot of exercise?" I asked.

"The books I have studied say that it is not necessary to knead yeast breads made from whole wheat flour. But if someone wants to knead the dough, there is no harm done and in fact the final result may produce a bread that has a finer texture and is less dense than nonkneaded whole wheat dough."

"How do you knead dough?" I asked.

"The most common way is to use the heel of your hand, or the heels of both hands and punch the dough again and again. This usually does not take more than about five minutes, after which the dough is dropped into an oiled pan and allowed to rise until it has about doubled in size.

"The rising of the dough may take about an hour. The dough should be kept in a draft-free place while it is rising and the temperature should be between 75° and 85°. Sometimes, I will place the dough to rise in a slightly heated oven, just warm enough for the warmth to be felt.

"I start preheating the oven about 10 minutes before I am ready to put in the bread. I will heat the oven to 350°. The bread will be ready in about 50 minutes, and there you have my favorite recipe for my favorite bread."

"Thanks, Evelyn," I replied. "I know that many people will be interested in your herbal health bread and I am sure that it will do them a lot of good and help them break the white flour bread habit."

DESSERTS FOR THE EVENING MEAL

This chapter is devoted to discussions of the evening meal. Now that we have discussed salads as well as preparation of bread, poultry, meats and fish, it is time to talk about desserts.

This is a sensitive subject to dieters. Many a good diet has been ruined because of the need to satisfy the "sweet tooth." Actually, there is no sweet tooth. Rather, there is a yearning for nourishment, due to improper food habits. Once the body gets the nutrients it needs, on a daily basis, there will be no such desire for sweets that causes so many dieters to depart from their diets.

However, for the benefit of so many readers accustomed to desserts, there are ways of overcoming the dessert problem, which we will now explore.

Nothing is better than a dessert of raw fruits. Cut up apples, pears, oranges, pineapple, strawberries, melons, watermelon, bananas or any other delicious fruits and make a fruit bowl for dessert. Sprinkle with some mint leaves for the herbal effect.

Many pies on the market have fruits, and sometimes a careless dieter will purchase a pie on the theory that fruit is fruit and so why not eat a delicious apple pie instead of some pieces of raw apple. Just one piece of apple pie (one-eighth of a nine-inch pie) would add 300 calories to the body whereas an entire large apple would add a total of only 80 calories—a difference well worth noting.

A piece of raisin pie would add 320 calories and a piece of pecan pie would add 430 calories. It's not the fruit alone that does it. It's the sugar, flavoring and fatty pie crust that causes the trouble.

There is no need to add into the fruit bowl all of the fruits that you can find. One or two would be enough. Often one fruit would do just fine, such as cantaloupe, strawberry or watermelon.

My own favorite dessert is to soak some prunes in the refrigerator overnight. I then have a fine cool prune juice drink. I will then take the softened prunes, place them in a bowl and add some yogurt or sour cream with some mint leaves. I often squeeze some fresh lemon over the prunes, just for the taste of it.

The gelatin desserts are also great favorites. For well over a hundred years, gelatin has been found to be an excellent food (not merely a desert) for persons recovering from an illness or those with troubled digestive systems.

The most common method of preparation of a gelatin dessert is to dissolve a heaping tablespoonful of the powdered gelatin into a pint of boiling water. Stir well and then remove from the heat and allow the gelatin mixture to cool down a little. You can then add sliced bananas, seedless grapes, strawberries, cantaloupe or any of a number of other fruits. Pour into a bowl and set into refrigerator for cooling.

Gelatin desserts lend themselves to an innumerable variety of combinations of fruits and herbs. In addition to fruits, you may want to try adding one or two of the following herbs: allspice, anise, caraway, cardamom seeds, chives, cinnamon, ginger, mace, nutmeg, poppy seeds, sesame seeds, spearmint (or other mint) leaves, thyme and vanilla.

Herbs and spices not only make foods tastier but also do their share in completing the day's nutritional requirements for vitamins and minerals. In addition, they also provide enzymes, fats, carbohydrates, protein and even hormones.

The downfall of most people, from the health viewpoint, is that they neglect each day to provide the body with the nutrients that are needed. Food should be prepared and selected daily with the view of meeting the daily nutritional requirements.

A deep concern for your health does not necessarily mean avoidance of pies, cakes, cookies and candies. It is entirely a matter of selection of the proper ingredients and avoidance of sugar and fattening foods as well as toxic substances. The result is a satisfaction of inner cravings long established by years of pleasurable but nevertheless improper living.

Pies are not necessarily dangerous to the overweight if a few precautions are taken. First, avoid recipes containing sugar and instead substitute some honey or blackstrap molasses. Use finely ground whole wheat flour instead of white flour. You may want to make a number of pie crusts at a time, even before you have any fillings for them. Make the crusts and roll them out into pie plates. Pile them on top of each other, with waxed paper between each plate and place them in the freezer to await the fillings. Make a dozen at a time, or half a dozen if you have a small family.

Here is a recipe for a single pie crust. For two crusts, you may double the recipe, etc. Take one cup of whole wheat flour, or pastry flour if you can get it, and combine in a bowl with one cup of wheat germ. If wheat germ is hard to get, use two cups of whole wheat flour or whole wheat pastry flour.

Add to the bowl one tablespoonful of blackstrap molasses or one tablespoonful of honey. Add one-half cup of corn oil, cold-pressed sesame seed oil or, if these items are not easily available, use safflower oil or some other low cholesterol oil. Add about three tablespoonfuls of cold water.

Blend all of the ingredients together. If too wet, add more flour; if too dry, add more water. When of a good solid consistency but pliable, move the mixture into a slightly oiled ten-inch pie plate.

After preheating the oven to 325°, bake for about 30 minutes (without any filling) until the pie crust is slightly brown and testing with a fork indicates that the crust is no longer soft or moist.

After the pie crust is ready, you are ready to drop the filling in. You then have a choice of immediately serving the hot pie crust with the filling or allowing the pie crust to cool off for a while and then placing the pie into the freezer, where it may be kept for several weeks until ready for use.

The best part of the pie is, of course, the filling. But you must be careful to select the proper ingredients. The fruits are the most delicious pie fillings and often some fruit combinations will make the pie even more delicious. Here again, a warning is necessary. Resist the temptation to add sugar. The fruits are naturally sweet but if you must sweeten, use honey.

While baking a pie does not destroy all the minerals or vitamins, there is general agreement that much of the life of the fruit, known as enzymes, are preserved during the freezing process but are destroyed during the process of baking. That is why I recommend that the pie crust be first baked and then the pie filling added to the crust after baking.

Pie fillings can vary from the simple to the sublime. The most simple is taking the fruit, washing it, removing the core, if it is an apple, and then cutting, chopping or slicing the fruit into small pieces or slices. That, itself, can be the filling and represents the ultimate in simplicity. If the fruit is apricot, peach, plum or cherry, the pits should also be removed.

If you want to make an upper crust, put it on over the filling and press the edges together. Take a fork and make a few openings over the crust so that the steam may escape. If you are going to have an upper crust, however, you will need to bake both the crusts and the filling as well. If you do, you will lose the vitamins that are destroyed by heat as well as the enzyme value.

While the bare fruit itself is a filling that should be not only delicious but healthy, a number of items may be added to the filling that will make it both tastier and healthier. For example, it is quite common to add raisins to the apples, pears, apricots or other fruits. Lemon juice is often added to the filling and the use of honey is not only desirable but practically a necessity if you are going to keep the fruit in a raw condition. Honey acts as a preservative. If the honey used is unheated and unfiltered, it not only contains vitamins, minerals and enzymes but also contains pollen, which is often sold separately as a food well supplied with protein, vitamins and minerals.

Incidentally, the unbaked pie fillings may themselves be used as a dessert, without having to be placed into a baked pie crust. To add to the taste, sprinkle some cinnamon, ginger, nutmeg, sesame seeds or mint leaves (chopped) over the filling.

Just as you have already seen that you need not deprive yourself of the joy of eating pie, you will be delighted to learn that you can eat cake, cookies and candy also. It all depends on the ingredients.

Instead of white flour, use whole wheat flour. Instead of sugar, use honey, maple syrup or molasses. Instead of chocolate, use carob. Instead of milk, use buttermilk. Instead of cream cheese, use sour cream or yogurt. You can take almost any recipe for cake and with a few minor changes you can produce a healthy food.

You can even have live enzymes with your baked cake by simply adding fresh fruit over the cake when it is served. The delights of delicious eating are not denied to the health enthusiast, where there is a will to find a way.

If you like chocolate cake, how would you like to eat a cake that looks like chocolate cake and tastes like chocolate cake but has no chocolate and no sugar and keeps the calories down to a minimum?

Powdered carob is a well-known substitute for chocolate. In fact, it tastes and looks so much like chocolate that many people cannot tell the difference. Instead of sugar, you may substitute pure maple syrup, honey or molasses. Try making a small cake at first, experimenting with the amount of carob or sweetener you would like.

You might try taking about two cups of whole wheat flour, un-bleached, and keep the flour ready for use. Into a blender, place one cup water and add one-half cup of buttermilk, two eggs, one teaspoonful of baking soda, a teaspoonful of vanilla and four tablespoonfuls of carob powder. After this is well blended, pour the mixture into a large bowl and add one-half cup of melted vegetable shortening. If you are not too worried about your fat intake, you may want to use unsalted butter instead of the shortening. Now is the time to add the sweetener, be it honey, molasses or maple syrup. A half cup is enough for sweetening but if you really want to make it very sweet, better make it a full cup.

Slowly add the whole wheat flour into the bowl, blend it together well and it is ready for the baking pan. You will probably want to divide the mixture into two pans, so that you can have an upper and lower layer with a special low-calorie frosting between the layers and over the outside of the cake. Of course, the frosting is applied after the two cakes are baked at about 400° for a period of 20 or 30 minutes. Jab a fork or knife into the cake and if there is wetness on the utensil when it is withdrawn, it's probably not yet ready. Be sure that the oven is preheated to the temperature you need before you place the cake into the oven.

Here's how to make the frosting: mix together about one-quarter cup of carob powder with a cup of powdered milk, one-quarter cup of honey, a teaspoonful of vanilla and two tablespoonfuls of melted butter.

Don't be tempted to use baking chocolate rather than carob. Remember that chocolate, from the cocoa bean, is high in cholesterol, calories, carbohydrates, fats and cocaine. Chocolate lacks nutritive value and is reported to deprive the body of nutrients. Chocolate contains oxalic acid, said to interfere with the ability of the body to absorb calcium.

On the other hand, carob is low in fat and rich in protein, calcium, natural carbohydrates and potassium. In addition, there are small quantities of sodium and iron to be found in carob, derived from pods of the carob tree. Other nutrients include the B vitamins and pectin.

To make your own carob powder, soak in hot water until soft and cut along the seam to open. Remove the seeds, cut the pod into small pieces and dry in a food dehydrator, oven or hot sun. After the pieces are dry, run the pieces through a grinder or blender several times and you then have the powder.

Another cake to try producing is the popular carrot cake. It's really not difficult! The hardest part is grating the carrots. The old-fashioned grating tool requires only a few minutes of time and there are many types of food processors on the market that do the job even quicker. My own favorite method is to use a juicer, make the juice and then mix the pulp and juice together for a rich carrot cake ingredient. Other times, I will use the carrot juice as a drink and use the pulp for either a carrot cake or a bread mix. For each two cups of grated carrots, use three cups of whole wheat flour. Use honey for sweetening, instead of sugar and use one egg for each cup of flour. Add one cup of vegetable oil for each cup of flour as well as a teaspoonful of baking powder with a teaspoonful of baking soda to each cup of flour.

Many cooks will add some chopped dates, nuts or raisins to the mixture and of course a teaspoonful or two of cinnamon and nutmeg enhances the flavor. Try to prevent the mixture from becoming too watery or too thick. You may want to add some crushed pineapple, orange juice, crushed apricots or other fruit. If the mixture appears to be too watery, add some more flour; if too thick, add some water or juice.

Also keep in mind the use of melted butter instead of vegetable oil and instead of honey, you may want to try maple syrup.

The oven should be preheated to 350° F for 30 minutes to an hour, depending upon the ingredients. A good baker watches the coloring of the cake (or bread or cookies). Once the product in the oven starts to turn brown, this is a sign of sufficient baking and another sign is the smell of food burning.

The same mixture used for making a carob or carrot cake may also be used for baking cookies. Simply use an oiled cookie sheet (flat baking dish) on which you drop about a tablespoonful of the mixture. The oven should be preheated to about 370° F and it usually takes from 10 to 12 minutes.

For cookies with spice, add ground cloves (about one-half teaspoonful) or the same amount of ground ginger to a basic cookie mix of two cups of whole wheat flour, an egg, a cup of honey or maple syrup.

There are some who may find fault with a diet book designed to produce weight reductions that deal with eating pies, cakes and cookies. However, it must be borne in mind that it is not so much the name of the food but rather it is the ingredients that matter. Pie fillings made of fresh fruits that have been frozen are really not to be compared to ordinary pies.

Nor are cakes or cookies made with whole wheat flour, without sugar, in the same class as cakes or cookies sold in stores or bakeries.

Another consideration is the need for permanence in weight loss. I would rather see an individual go on a diet that allowed an occasional piece of pie for dessert, with a piece of wholesome cake or cookies and an herb tea during a period of relaxation, than for a person to go on a diet for a week or two and then go back to the sugar, fat and white flour life because of an unwillingness to forego forever the joys of desserts.

The word "candy" may cause a diet book censor to frown but not when the so-called candy is composed of combinations of fruits and honey.

For your children or for yourself, an occasional honey-dipped dried fruit will satisfy the desire for sweets and at the same time allow the dieter to eat sensibly.

To make homemade candied fruits, take the fruit and either cut into half or into smaller pieces as desired. For example, apricots, pears and whole figs, if not of enormous size, may be cut in half but larger fruit such as apples, peaches and pineapple should be cut into smaller pieces. Cherries may be dried whole as people know that a cherry is likely to contain a pit and will watch for it during the chewing process. For the more fastidious, the cherry may be either sliced or pierced with a knife and the pit removed.

Whatever fruit you want to candy-dry, first wash and peel it if necessary, as with oranges. Drop the fruit into boiling water for not more than five minutes and then drain. Incidentally, the water can be placed in jars in the refrigerator and used later as a cool and refreshing drink instead of plain water.

In a separate pot, boil for 15 minutes three-quarters of a cup of water and one pound of honey for each pound of fruit. For example, if you have two pounds of fruit, use two pounds of honey and one and one-half cups of water. Then pour the honey-water, after it has been boiled, over the fruit, and boil the whole mixture for about 15 minutes. Remove it from the fire and allow it to cool for about seven hours. Most cooks allow it to stand overnight. The process of boiling for 15 minutes and allowing to stand overnight is repeated for five nights, after which time all of the syrup is absorbed into the fruit. The fruit is then removed from the syrup and allowed to dry in the sun or in a dehydrator. Honey is known to have lasted for hundreds of years without spoiling and when absorbed into a sweet fruit in the manner explained the fruit takes on the character of the honey and will retain the freshness of newly picked fruit.

And of course, you must not neglect to use herbs and spices for flavoring of various fruits. For berries, use cinnamon, clove, ginger, nutmeg, rosemary or vanilla for flavoring. For apricots or peaches, use allspice, cinnamon, cloves, ginger, nutmeg, rosemary or almond extract. Try sprinkling lightly over the candied fruits when ready for serving. For cherries, try allspice, cloves, cinnamon, mace, mint or nutmeg and for pineapple, try allspice, cardamom, cinnamon, cloves, coriander, mace, mint, nutmeg, rosemary or vanilla flavoring. If you have made some strawberry candy, try sprinkling with allspice, cinnamon, cloves, or rosemary.

Chapter Nine

How the Herbal Diet
Program
Prevents Backsliding

He who is convinced against his will is of the same opinion still.

Author unknown

IN this chapter, as in other chapters, an open mind is vitally important. If you are doubtful at the very start that herbs can help you, before you even try them, you have fallen into a psychological trap that can wreck your weight-losing program.

Please keep an open mind about the herbal diet. Once you are convinced that it can help, you will want to use it to change any undesirable eating habits you may have.

The herbal diet is ideal to prevent the return to bad eating habits, known as backsliding, because herbs lend a taste and tang to foods otherwise looked down upon as bland and lacking the luster and attraction of the so-called "convenience" foods.

In addition to the taste and fragrance of appetizing herbs, the ability of herbs to activate various glands and organs of the body is well known. As a result, the herbal diet becomes an exciting diet that attracts and holds like a strong magnet.

AVOIDING TRAPS THAT CAUSE BACKSLIDING OFF THE DIET

Backsliding is often the result of partaking of products containing sugar. These products include not only soft drinks, candies, ice cream, cookies, cake, pie, donuts and the sugared breakfast cereals but also the more subtle refined carbohydrates found in most comercial breads, canned fruits, orange juice, jellies, custards and even fresh sweet fruits.

Despite the common belief that fruits cannot hurt you but may be eaten without restriction, some of the dried as well as fresh fruits contain large quantities of sugar in the form of carbohydrates. Even honey, long admired by many as an excellent sugar substitute, contains about 80 percent levulose and dextrose, both of which are forms of sugar.

Another popular misconception is that the body's nutritional requirements make the intake of carbohydrates essential to the body's well-being. This may be true when an individual is underweight but when there is excessive fatty tissue, the need of the body for carbohydrates is met by conversion of fat into sugar. To state it bluntly, the overweight person should omit carbohydrates from the diet if he or she wants to get rid of that excessive fat. Find out which foods are high in carbohydrate content and avoid them.

To avoid traps that cause backsliding, you must first recognize the trap when you see it. Carbohydrates in seemingly harmless form such as whole wheat bread are nevertheless carbohydrates, and consuming whole wheat bread or other carbohydrates does not help the serious dieter to overcome his or her excessive weight problem.

Another trap that causes backsliding is the consumption of excessive amounts of protein on the theory that as protein is not fat and also it is not a carbohydrate it is therefore harmless to the body. Actually, excessive protein, not required for bodily needs, is converted by the body's chemical processes into sugar, in one form or another.

While sugar is definitely needed by the body, it is the *excessive quantity* that must be avoided! Sugar does provide energy but if your intake of sugar or some other carbohydrate is greater than what is needed or consumed it is stored in the body and oversaturates the blood with a high sugar content. Eating or drinking more than is needed causes excessive weight increase.

THE CALORIE CATASTROPHY

Excessive calories are catastrophic to the body chemistry. In addition to sugar and products containing sugar, calories are carried to the body in the form of foods prepared with fatty acids. One of the chief carriers of fat, so often disguised as palatable foods, is the fried food product. While the potato, for example, is a good food product, combining it with fat, in the process of deep frying, makes the potato a carrier of fat, difficult to digest and adding sharply to body weight. The same applies to any fish that is deep fried.

Some people think that it is only deep fried food that is dangerous. Actually, food that is fried with only a small amount of fat is even more dangerous than food that is deep fried. The reason for this is that in addition to saturating the food with fat, a small amount of fat is subjected to higher heat than deep fried fat, because of the close contact with the extremely hot surface of the pan. The great heat intensity converts what was merely a dangerous fatty food to a toxic poisonous substance that is not only indigestible but represents a dangerous hazard to the glands and organs of the body.

It's time that we thoroughly understood calories. A calorie is only a measurement of energy. You consume food and it turns into energy. The amount of energy used is measured in terms of calories. The amount of food consumed is measured in calories. If the amount of energy used equals the amount of calories consumed, then there is an equalization of food consumed with energy expended and all is well, provided that you have the ideal weight. If you are overweight, your energy supply generated by the food you consume must not be larger than the amount of energy expended by exercise, recreation, walking or just plain breathing. (There is muscular action involved in the inhalation and exhalation of breath that consumes energy or calories.)

AVOIDING TEMPTATION

Any minister will tell you that if you want to keep from sinning, stay away from temptation. The same rule applies if you want to avoid the temptations of fattening foods. Change to a diet of consuming only unprocessed fresh foods as much as possible. There are many tasty foods that can be prepared without the need for eating processed foods, especially if herbs and spices are used to give a pleasant fragrance and spicy taste to the foods and drinks. It can be done!

There are many sweet and delicious foods such as sweet potatoes, yams and carrots. Freshly made carrot juice is especially sweet and delicious as a drink and is highly nourishing and rich with vitamin A.

Avoid drinking processed milk, caffeine-filled coffee or tea or soft drinks loaded with caffeine or other toxic substances. Try replacing such drinks with herb teas such as mint, alfalfa, comfrey, sage, elder, violet, harrow, ginseng, camomile, pepper grass, witchgrass, sassafras root and dozens of other teas. The teas just mentioned are especially recommended for people desiring to lose excessive weight and are obtainable from almost any good health food store. A little honey may be added to the cup of tea for sweetening and a slice of lemon always adds to the flavor.

Avoid the temptation of banned foods and drinks by not buying them and not having them close by when a desire arises. This rule is especially true when you awake in the middle of the night with a feeling of hunger. If the wrong food is in the refrigerator, the temptation may be too much to withstand and your diet program goes down the drain.

Unless some serious chronic illness is present, which may require the services of a physician, herbalists recommend the herb known as passion flower for a sedative. Make a tea out of it before going to bed at night and the chances are good that you will have a sound sleep. It is not habit forming.

OFFICER LEN S. AND HIS SNACKING HABIT

Officer Len S. had been warned by his sergeant that he was overweight and that he had better get on a diet. It seems that Len was afflicted with "snackitis." He was always getting a snack and this had ruined his physique.

His weight of 220 pounds was too much for his height of five feet seven inches. Len had a serious problem. He needed to be taught how to convert the snacking habit into a good habit.

Len was told about three plants that helped him reduce. For snacking, he started carrying two thermos bottles with him, one filled with prune juice and the other with fig juice, both good laxatives and yet not drastic in action. He carried a third plant in powder form—a product of the sea known as kelp. Herbalists recommend kelp highly for reducing obesity. It is available in powdered form and Len was told to sprinkle it on all of his foods, including the prune and fig juices.

When Len became hungry for a snack, he drank a little prune juice or fig juice with kelp. His hunger lessened and after a week on this program, he had gotten rid of his snacking habit.

A SYSTEM FOR 2 PERCENT WEIGHT LOSS WEEKLY

Herbs can help you in systematic weight reduction without backsliding but you must establish reasonable goals. A weight loss of 2 percent each week is not too much or too little. For example, if you weigh 200 pounds, a 2 percent weight loss would be 4 pounds a week. In ten weeks, 40 pounds can be lost without any drastic measures such as fasting, although fasting under supervision of a nutritionist would not be dangerous

You will need to keep close count of your weight losses and gains, if any. Get a sheet of paper and draw some vertical and horizontal lines on it. Show your weight on the first day of the program and each day show your new weight. Don't be discouraged if you gain a little on one day or another.

Determine the amount of weight loss that you want to achieve and decide, first of all, to select good foods that will give you balanced nutrition. Remember that your diet should contain all of the necessary protein, vitamins, minerals, carbohydrates and fats that your body needs but not more than what your body needs.

You should not have to return to old food habits for fear of illness so long as you eat a well-balanced diet. One important fact, often overlooked, is that the stomach, intestines and bowels have become overdistended due to prolonged stretching from overeating for many years. Consequently, there may be a feeling of emptiness for a while but as you get used to the feeling of slenderness and realize that your body should be given only the quantities that it needs and not given as much food as it can take, the fear of illness or death from starvation will go away.

Another popular misconception is that food needs to be cooked to be palatable. I believe in food preparation, but this does not necessarily mean cooking. Of course, it all depends upon the food. If it is a food that requires cooking in order for it to be tenderized, then cooking is all right. But remember that cooking in water usually results in most of the nutrients going into the water. When potatoes are cooked in water, for example, the water itself becomes a nourishing drink due to the loss of nutrients from potatoes into the water. A baked potato retains the nutrients in the potato. Likewise, broiled foods are better than boiled foods, and, of course, frying of foods should be avoided altogether.

You should select foods for a double purpose; choose both those that are enjoyable and those that provide the necessary nutrients needed by your body. Do not worry about not getting enough. A few mouthfuls of any food is usually enough. The main thing to remember is to eat a variety of nutrients so that you get all the vitamins, minerals, protein, carbohydrates and fat that your body needs. For those who already have enough fat, this may be omitted from the diet. Carbohydrates, such as bread and potatoes, may also be omitted from the diet so long as the body can draw from the supply that has been stored. If you feel some hunger, that is a good sign because it shows that your body will now start drawing from the excessive supply you have in storage.

Start the day with a good breakfast. Buy yourself two bananas, two peaches and two grapefruit. Stock your kitchen with a dozen large eggs and a loaf of whole wheat bread. You will have enough food then for at least six days of breakfasts. By confining your breakfast to one slice of toast and two eggs, followed with one piece of fruit, you will take in a large variety of food nutrients. To make the breakfast more interesting and thus prevent backsliding, sprinkle some herbs on your eggs. You will find that adding herbs and spices to your foods will add a tang to your meals that will make your diet interesting and will be an inducement for you to maintain it.

To have enough lunches for a week, buy two small cans of tuna fish, two cans of salmon and two of sardines. These will give you variety and, more importantly, the protein and other nutrients your body will need during your diet. Get a head of lettuce, three or four tomatoes, about two large onions, an avocado or two and a variety of season fresh fruits, enough for consuming two a day. If you get grapes, plums or other small fruit, buy one pound for the week.

For lunch, each day you should open a small can of tuna fish, salmon or sardines, toast some whole wheat bread (two slices), and make yourself two open-faced sandwiches. Bread does not really need a spread, but if habit makes you feel you must have a spread, use the avocado and spread it over the bread. Place a slice of tomato on the bread and cover it with a slice of onion. Spread some of the fish of your choice over the onion and cover with a leaf of lettuce. By preparing two open-faced sandwiches (one with each slice of bread), you will have a well-rounded lunch with practically all of the vitamins and minerals that the body needs. For a more rapid rate of reducing weight, omit the bread.

To purchase food for your dinners, get a supply of six or seven servings of fish or meat per person in your family, whichever meat you prefer. If you are a vegetarian, you can omit fish and meat from your diet and you may want, instead, to buy and consume more vegetables to replace the protein that you would obtain from fish or meat. Alfalfa and bean sprouts are protein-rich vegetables. Some vegetarians also avoid dairy products of every type, including eggs. If you are a vegetarian, eat soybeans and soybean products to get your proteins. Nuts and seeds are also good protein sources but unfortunately they are also rich in fats.

When preparing your dinner, be sure to broil, not fry, the fish or meat that you may prepare. The process of frying creates intense heat, especially when the food is browned. Frying food will often produce toxic elements that are ingested into the system and result in all kinds of health problems, including the danger of cancer. Avoid trouble by cooking without frying. A bit of lettuce (or celery) with a slice of toasted whole wheat bread should provide sufficient nutrients for dinner to go with the fish or meat. Don't forget to sprinkle the foods freely with herbs such as garlic or red pepper. I have already mentioned kelp as a good herb for sprinkling on foods; others are garlic, red pepper, oregano and parsley. There are many more. Some firms have placed some herb combinations in small glass jars with sprinkler tops for handy use. Read the labels carefully, because there may be a temptation on the part of some herb distributors to add table salt to herb combinations, or they may use chemical preservatives that should generally be avoided.

There is enough food in this program for a continuing weight loss weekly without danger of insufficient nutrition. To lose 2 percent weekly, avoid drinking coffee, milk or other liquids with meals. Generally speaking, all food has a high percentage of water already, so that there is no need to drink water or other liquids with meals. If you must drink, make some orange juice from natural oranges (not the artificial flavors or even frozen) or some grapefruit juice. Prune juice is great for keeping bowel movements regular.

OVERCOMING COMPULSIONS FOR FOOD

Tom C. loves to eat. Even during reducing and afterwards, he still loves to eat. However, he has learned to control his appetite. He used to eat as much as he could but not now. Now that he has learned to control his eating habits, he loves to eat even more than before but he had learned to eat only enough for his bodily needs.

Learning when to stop eating had not been easy for Tom. He had always thought it was only necessary to fill his stomach, no matter with what. He had been raised in a low income family and food was not plentiful during his days of growing up. Now that he was in a position to buy all the food he wanted, he splurged and gained in weight well above his actual needs.

The course of treatment included an education in nutrition. He was taught the importance and need for vitamins, minerals, proteins, carbohydrates and fats in the body. He gradually realized that although the quantity had to be adequate, it was the quality and nutritive value of the food that mattered.

To keep from backsliding, Tom was taught how to use herbs and spices to make the food more attractive. The result was that he became greatly attracted to broiled fish and steaks, flavored well with exotic herbs and spices. His weight went down, he feels fine and he still loves food.

DANGERS OF THE COFFEE BREAK

The so-called "coffee break" may be around for a long while. The spurt of energy received from the drinking of coffee, which stimulates the heart and speeds up blood circulation for a while, has dangerous aspects. Few people know, unfortunately, that excessive coffee, due to the presence of about 100 milligrams of caffeine in a strong cup of coffee, may cause palpitation of the heart, trembling, nervousness, insomnia, anxiety and general depression.

It is well known that when anyone sits down for a cup of coffee, it is not only the coffee that is swallowed. It is usually "coffee and." The "and" is often a sweet roll, a donut or even a sandwich. There is something about coffee that makes you hungry and of course the more you eat the heavier you get. Coffee also disturbs the digestion of many people and they try to protect themselves by eating something with every cup. This, too, leads to overweight conditions.

Yes, there are alternatives to the coffee break. Ginseng tea is the front runner. It is not only a general stimulant, giving the "lift" so badly wanted but has several other benefits, including relief for headaches and back pains.

Another good substitute for the coffee break is the use of the herb known as hibiscus. Rich in vitamin C, this herb has an attractive taste with a pleasing red color. The high vitamin content is believed to be effective for preventing colds and influenza.

Once the coffee break habit is conquered, with its accompanying food binges, you will not want to backslide into the old bad eating and drinking habits.

HOW HARRY H. COPED WITH HUNGER PANGS

Harry H. had tried several diet programs but after he lost some weight he would backslide into his bad eating habits. He explained that he would get some strong hunger pangs and he would get frightened that something would happen to him if he did not take care of those hunger pangs.

Again, it is largely a matter of education. The body needs only certain nutrients to keep going. After these nutrients are supplied, any extra foods or food substitutes put into the stomach simply makes extra work for the digestive system and, if the food is not needed, it is stored away in the body as fat. Even protein is converted into fat during the body metabolic processes if there is already sufficient protein present.

As the manager of a large supermarket, Harry had no problem about his selection of foods, which he obtained with his employee discount. He could afford choice cuts of meat, fish or anything else. His big dieting problem was his wife. Not intentionally, of course, but she did manage to tempt his appetite with delicious foods that she knew he enjoyed. She was proud that she provided Harry with delicious meals. Unfortunately, she did not realize that dieters can enjoy their food too.

In meetings with Harry, he seemed to be knowledgeable of the principles of basic nutrition but he compared his wife to a large steamship headed in a certain direction. It would take some doing to get her to change her direction. Although Harry discussed the problem with his wife on several occasions, it was no use. All she did was to make the meals more delicious and appetizing so as to stop his complaining.

What could poor Harry do? He was in a dilemma! On the one hand, he had his wife, his marriage and those delicious but fattening meals. On the other hand, he had his health and longevity to think of. He was already 54 years of age and knew of some younger friends who were overweight and who had fatal heart attacks, probably brought about by the carrying of extra weight and blocking of the arteries by congestion with substances that accumulate in the arteries because of wrong ingestion of foods. The big question! Should he go along with his wife and take a chance on a long life despite his being overweight or should he follow the good nutrition program that he knew he should follow for good health?

The solution? A compromise. He continued to eat the food his wife prepared but ate only one-half or less of the previous portions. In addition, he sprinkled various herbs liberally over the food he ate, such as hawthorn, red pepper, garlic and hibiscus. He found that his hunger pangs disappeared when he ate less food copiously sprinkled with a variety of herbs and spices. Also, he ate more slowly and relished each mouthful. He chewed his food thoroughly, masticating each mouthful until it turned into a liquid, thereby easing the digestive processes.

When questions came from his wife as to why the herbs, he had his answers ready. The hawthorn was for the heart, to help it to carry the heavier load of overweight and to help clear the arteries; the red pepper was a heart stimulant that worked in a gentle and harmless way and the garlic improved the kidney function. The hibiscus tea drink, being heavily loaded with vitamin C, helped to prevent colds and influenza.

The expected counter-questions came, of course! What heart condition? What kidney trouble? What infection? Harry had been carefully coached as to the answers. He told her that the best way to combat disease was to prevent it. He explained to her the danger of a high-calorie food intake program; how heavy eating endangered the heart, the kidneys and in fact all parts of the body. The strain could easily weaken the body and reduced resistance causes colds, influenza and disease of all kinds.

The final outcome was that Harry's wife reconsidered her position about dieting, fattening foods were taken off the household menu, herb teas were added and both Harry and his wife are now eating properly and feeling fine.

SATISFYING THE SWEET TOOTH

"Sweet tooth" really means a feeling or desire for energy. Some people get that energy when they eat a candy bar, drink some soda pop or a cup of coffee. Others like to eat a cookie, some cake, donuts or pastry. This all comes under the heading of satisfying the sweet tooth.

There are some herbs that act as stimulants and, when taken, should supply as much energy or more than any of the aforementioned foods or drinks. These herbs include peppermint, cayenne (red pepper), cloves, horseradish and black pepper.

To use these tasty and spicy herbs without first embarking upon a good diet program would not make good sense. Good health and a feeling of well-being does not result merely from the use of herbs, just as good health does not result from the use of sweets. Just as a drunk believes that his salvation lies in obtaining another good drink of whiskey, so does the junk food addict think that another cup of coffee or a candy bar is all that is needed.

Sometimes change is hard to accomplish. There is a law in physics that an object in action tends to remain in action just as an object at rest tends to remain at rest. After years of bad eating and drinking habits, it is often difficult for a person to change; however, it is often a case of diet or die and there are only a few persons who are willing to take chances with their lives. Having eaten meat, potatoes and gravy for many years, with white bread, beer, wine and alcoholic beverages, it is a small miracle to produce any changes. However, it can be done. Education is the strongest power for accomplishing changes of this kind.

Peppermint leaves soaked in either hot or cold water and combined with some lemon juice and honey makes a sweet drink that not only satisfies the sweet tooth but is generally recognized as having beneficial effects. Peppermint serves as a stimulant and tonic and also removes gas from the stomach and intestines.

SUBSTITUTES FOR DESSERT

One of the main reasons for backsliding is the memory of delicious apple pie smothered with whipped cream or chocolate cake with ice cream. Why go on a diet and deprive yourself of such delightful occasions? There are other healthful foods that can be substituted for calorie-rich foods that provide energy not needed and are therefore stored away in the hips or other parts of the body.

A fruit bowl of pieces of melon, apple, banana, pear and other fruit is just about as tasty a morsel as any other food. At the same time, there is no buildup of fat or excessive energy.

Tropical fruits such as pineapple, papaya and coconuts are especially delicious dessert foods. Instead of whipped cream, try sprinkling some powdered herbs and spices on fruit desserts. The result will be a most interesting taste and plenty of energy to make you feel fine.

WHAT SUSY R. DID DURING "TRYING" DIET PERIODS

Susy R., after much deliberation and carefully considering her over-weight condition, decided to go on a diet. She was 50 pounds overweight, all gained after a recent pregnancy. She told me frankly that she was not sure whether or not she could maintain the diet when started as she had a strong liking for good food tastily prepared.

One of the things to do during periods of temptation to go off the diet is to eat grapes. They are fine for cleansing the body internally, usually readily available in the markets and yield quickly the energy sought by someone tempted to go off a good diet program. After being told it was all right to eat grapes, Susy did quite well in maintaining her diet program.

THE HERBAL DIET REDUCING CLUB

One of the best ways to keep from backsliding is to belong to a diet club where diet problems are discussed. Better yet is the herbal diet club, where members study the use of herbs in dieting. If there is no herbal diet club in your area, start one.

It may be best to first start a herbal society to learn about herbs and to then include diet studies within the herbal society. One reason for this procedure is that many persons are sensitive in connection with weight problems and would prefer to be simply a member of an herbal society rather than be a member of a weight reduction club.

First, ask the local public library if there is a small meeting room available without charge to organize an herbal society and to hold meetings there. If the public library does not have such a meeting room, there may be a local high school auditorium available.

Second, after arrangements are made for the place of the meeting, secure a speaker to discuss herbs, dieting with herbs or a combination of both. There may even be a book review of the book you are now holding and in fact there may be a series of discussions based upon chapters of this book.

Third, members who are dieting should be encouraged to tell about their experiences, the food and liquids they are drinking and their successes in weight reduction. This not only informs nondieting members and encourages them to diet but by discussing their own problems members become encouraged and imbued with the desire to do what they say in public they will do. Incidentally, this is an important characteristic of many diet clubs. The members go to the meetings to report on their own individual progress with their diets as well as to listen to how other members are overcoming similar problems.

Chapter Ten

How to Slim Down
with Sprouts

Those who have the true wisdom remain strong, while those who have no wisdom grow old and feeble.

Old Chinese Saying
(Nei Ching)

THERE are many Chinese who believe in prevention rather than cure. In fact, many Chinese physicians will not undertake to treat the sick, comparing such treatment to the behavior of persons who begin to dig a well after they have become thirsty. They believe that illness comes only to those who violate basic rules of the universe and they see their function as teachers or educators of the people so that they will avoid disease.

THE SUPERIOR BENEFITS OF SPROUT EATING

Sprouts for reducing represents the epitome of any reducing diet. Not only are there practically all of the needed vitamins and minerals in sprouts but there is a complete absence of toxic substances on this vegetable food, not having been sprayed with insecticides while growing. Also, the fat content is practically nil and so here is a food that is free of cholesterol. In addition, testing with animals revealed that grain sprouts contain all of the necessary amino acids to constitute a complete protein.

Studies in President College, Calcutta, India revealed that sprouting produces choline, a lipotropic agent that apparently eliminates fatty tissue. Thus, with sprouts providing valuable nutrients and at the same time working to eliminate fat, the use of sprouts provides a double-edged weapon in the fight for a normal body weight.

At King's College, in England, experiments resulted in the finding that sprouts are better than lemon juice in the prevention and treatment of scurvy, the disease resulting from a lack of vitamin C in the diet. At McGill University, in Montreal, dried peas were sprouted and high levels of vitamin C were found, comparable to orange juice. Experiments at the University of Pennsylvania revealed that soybeans contained high levels of vitamin C and similar high levels of vitamin C were found in sprouting experiments with oats at the Kansas Agricultural Experiment Station. It has also been reported that sprouted wheat produces excellent results in the strengthening of bones. In addition to vitamin C, wheat sprouts contain vitamins B-1, B-2, niacin, pantothenic acid, pyridoxine, biotin, folic acid and, in common with all other sprouts, contain live enzymes, a highly valuable nutrient.

In addition to the remarkable benefits of sprouts, perhaps most valuable of all is the practical benefit of knowing that there can never be a problem as to soil conditions, drought, storms or other bad weather, insecticides (as there are no bug problems in sprouting) or storage. A new crop is ready every two or three days and one pound of seeds increases seven or eight-fold in quantity of food, making sprout seeds one of the most economical methods of beating the high cost of living.

At Yale University, sprouting experiments were conducted with many varieties of seeds, including oats, wheat, barley, corn, peas, buckwheat, limas and mung beans. The results verified the presence of valuable vitamins. In addition to the finding of vitamins A, B and C, sprouts have been found to be rich in vitamin E, a vitamin essential for good health. Incidentally, bean sprouts do not have the objectionable gas-generating quality of the whole bean so that it is just not the same as eating beans.

Another remarkable benefit of sprouts is the ease with which they can be stored. If you have too many, you can put them in the freezer and their nutritive values will be practically all retained. Even when dried in the sun or in a dehydrator, they retain their nutritive values.

Also, they can be used in practically all foods. Sprinkle some sprouts over a plate of soup, mix them with scrambled eggs, blend them into bakery products with the dough and see how much better the bread or rolls will taste. The Chinese use soybean and mung bean sprouts lavishly in their food preparations. Sprouts go well as an accompaniment to fruit desserts. For an additional treat, sprinkle with some sunflower seeds. An excellent drink is prepared by placing sprouts in a blender and liquefying them.

And of great interest to dieters, the enzymes in sprouts help you to digest and absorb the food you eat. Without adequate enzymes, the face and body starts to sag and wither and early aging starts, no matter the diet, the medication, the physicians or the hospitals.

I have already mentioned how university experiments in Calcutta revealed that sprouting produces choline. Other experiments, conducted at Auburn University, Alabama, have shown that a deficiency in choline, a vitamin in the B complex, caused test animals to develop cancer within a very short time. Thus, it is clear that generous portions of sprouts daily should be an important part of the daily diet.

GROWING YOUR OWN SPROUTS

The use of a wide-mouth fruit jar seems to be the easiest and most popular method of growing sprouts. If a fruit jar isn't handy, use any wide-mouth jar. You will need a strainer of some kind at the top of the jar so that you can keep the seeds moist, which will necessitate rinsing at least two or three times a day. The strainer will keep the seeds from being poured out with the water. There are sprouting jars on the market with metal strainers or, if you wish, you can make holes in the lid cover, large enough to allow the water to leave but not large enough for the seeds to escape when you do the rinsing.

Other forms of strainers are cheesecloth, held in place with a rubber band or some white nylon net, available in shops where dry goods are sold. If you use a fruit jar, you can use the same jar to store the sprouts in the refrigerator when they are ready to eat. In that case, you may use the original metal rim that came with the fruit jar at the time of purchase.

There are also some specially made and patented sprouting kits available from health food stores that may simplify the sprouting process for you, or you may want to experiment with some methods of your own. For example, one homemade method is to sprinkle the seeds over a towel, cover with another towel and allow a light shower of water (outdoors, of course) to run constantly over the towels. With this method, there is no need to rinse the seeds. The constant sprinkling will keep the seeds moist and allow them to grow. After sprouting starts, the upper towel should be removed to avoid obstruction of the growth.

For ideal sprouting, the water used should be free from chlorine or fluorine. Make sure that the seeds you buy are of high quality and that they will sprout. Ask the seller for assurance that they will sprout. When you get home, take a few seeds, soak them overnight and keep them moist and refreshed with clean, warm water several times a day for the next day or two to make sure the seeds sprout. If they do not, take your supply back to the seller and ask for a fresh supply of seeds that will sprout.

The quantity of sprouting seeds to place into a jar depends upon the size of the jar. A safe rule is to place enough seeds in to cover the bottom of the jar when it is upright.

The first step, after placing the seeds into the jar, is to allow the seeds to soak overnight, preferably in warm water, from 70° to 80° F. Some sprouters will first pour the seeds they plan to use into a flat dish so as to look them over and remove any stones or foreign objects that may have become mixed into the seed container. Also, cracked and broken seeds should be removed. It is also advisable to wash the seeds by rinsing in water before placing them into the jar or other receptacle for sprouting.

After the first soaking overnight of the washed seeds, the water is then drained out of the jar, the seeds rinsed with warm water and the water then allowed to drain out. It is good advice to save the water used in soaking overnight for drinking purposes or mixing with juices or soups. This water has been found to contain a fairly large quantity of water-soluble vitamins and minerals and should not be wasted.

Rinsing and draining should take place morning, noon and evening for ideal sprouting. As previously mentioned, it is best to use water that is without chlorine and without fluorine, found in many city water supplies. Depending upon the seeds used, sprouts may be ready to eat in two or three days.

There is a difference of opinion as to when to eat the sprouts; that is, when they first appear or after they have been allowed to grow several inches long. Some authorities say that the grain sprouts, such as wheat and rye, should be eaten when the sprout has grown as long as the original seed from whence it came. Of course, in such event, the sprout will be quite small. Others say that the sprouts should be allowed to grow to a length of several inches and that the little leaves that grow out from the wheat and alfalfa sprouts are especially tasty. It is customary, for maximum benefits, to eat the entire sprout complex, root, stem and clinging seed husks. Mung bean and soybean sprouts are often allowed to grow to three inches in height before being placed on the breakfast, luncheon or dinner table. They are fine for all meals. You can also liquefy sprouts for healthful drinking.

HOW ERNEST Z. BECAME A SPROUTARIAN

Ernest Z. weighed 280 pounds and didn't know what to do about it. He realized that for a man of his height, five feet, eight inches, his weight should be about 150 pounds. He had 130 pounds to lose. I informed him of the importance of obtaining all of the necessary vitamins, minerals, protein, carbohydrates and a small amount of fat each day.

However, I was rather surprised when he started our regular weekly consultation with the announcement that he had become a sproutarian.

"What made you become a sproutarian?" I asked. "If you will recall our conversations, at no time did I even mention the word to you."

"That's true," he admitted. "But you did advise me to beware of food that had been sprayed with insecticides. Well, sprouts are grown to eating size in about two or three days and in that short time, there is no chance for insects to take a hold; therefore they are not sprayed with insecticides or pesticides."

"Now, just a minute," I argued. "There's more to eating food than selecting food that has not been sprayed with insecticides."

Secretly, I was very pleased with the action of Ernest. Sprouts are very beneficial in many ways, but I wanted to see whether or not Ernest really knew of the value of sprouts or whether he was merely indulging in a passing fancy.

"Do you mean to say," Ernest inquired questioningly, "that you don't know the wonderful benefits of sprouting?"

"I know a few things about sprouts," I replied, "but what made you become a sproutarian?"

"As you know," Ernest replied, "it's always been easy for me to catch cold and I often forget to take my vitamins and oranges and lemons are not always available. Ever since I started on sprouts, I haven't had a cold because sprouts are rich in vitamin C. In fact, soybean sprouts are said to contain about eight times the amount of vitamin C in oranges or lemons."

"OK," I said. "So sprouts give you plenty of vitamin C. What else do you get from sprouts?"

"I did quite a lot of reading about sprouts. I learned that alfalfa, which ranchers know as ideal for livestock, also contains some very important amino acid proteins and at least eight essential enzymes required by the body for the digestion of food."

Ernest was right. The word alfalfa itself is of Arabic origin and means "father of all foods." The Arabs first experimented with alfalfa many years ago and the word spread until at the present time it is used practically everywhere.

"What else do you know about alfalfa?" I challenged.

Thus far, I was very pleased with Ernest. But how much did he really learn about alfalfa and other sprouts?

"In addition to vitamin C," Ernest replied, "alfalfa contains all of the vitamins. It even has vitamin K, needed by the body for clotting of the blood in case of a cut or other wound which might break a blood vessel."

"Are you going to tell me that alfalfa is a complete food?" I asked.

"There's no doubt about it. Not only does it have all the vitamins, most of the enzymes and the protein amino acids but scientists have found that alfalfa has potassium, phosphorus, calcium, magnesium, sodium, silicon and many more minerals needed by the body."

"Does being a sproutarian help you to lose weight?"

"At the rate I'm going, it will not be long before my overweight problem will be gone. I'm losing from one to three pounds almost daily and, best of all, I feel fine doing it."

Well, you just can't beat success. He had the knowledge and the willpower, which are probably the two most important ingredients in practically any formula for winning most of the battles of life.

HOW TO SPROUT YOUR OWN SALADS

Keep all kinds of seeds sprouting all of the time. In this way, you can be assured of a variety of sprouts in your sprout salad. Not only will you lose weight but doctor and hospital bills will be a thing of the past.

If you are using jars for sprouting, cover with cheesecloth or similar material that will allow you to rinse the water at least twice a day. Plan on using up the sprouts being grown in the bottle on the third day after starting them. If you start sprouts on a Monday, you may want to attach a label and mark it "Thursday." This means that the sprouts in this jar must be eaten on Thursday.

There is nothing wrong in mixing the seeds at the time of sprouting. In this way, you have your salad already mixed when you pour the sprouts into your dish.

Remember, too, that the seeds should be soaked overnight or all day long at the start of the sprouting period and this counts as one day. After the first day of soaking, there are really only two days for sprouting.

Some of the more popular sprouts are alfalfa, mung bean, wheat, rye, oat groats, soybean, sesame, sunflower and squash seeds. Pinto beans, chili beans, kidney beans and corn can also be easily sprouted, using the same procedure of soaking for one day and sprouting for two days. Garbanzo beans, lentils and peas may also be sprouted in the same way.

BEATRICE L. SERVES SPROUTARIAN LUNCHEONS

If you are ever invited to lunch at the home of Beatrice L., you will have the most delicious and healthiest lunch of your life.

Beatrice used to be a fatty. At five feet, seven inches tall, she weighed 170 pounds when I first met her. Her husband regarded her as pleasingly plump but they both had sense enough to know that being overweight could lead to all kinds of illnesses.

As with all cases where changing of food habits is necessary, it is always best to make the change gradually, following a program of education in the basics of nutrition. After attending some of my health lectures, Beatrice and her husband decided to switch to a program of quasi-vegetarianism. She was especially intrigued with the wonderful qualities of sprouts and learned to make some fascinating and tasteful sprout dishes.

One of her favorites would resemble a bird's nest. She would fashion the nest out of alfalfa sprouts and inside the "nest" she would arrange some sprouted peas, garbanzo beans and almonds. Over it all, she would sprinkle some lemon juice.

There is no limit to the combinations that may be tried for variety and taste. Mung bean sprouts may be substituted for the alfalfa sprouts and lentil sprouts, combined with sprouted onion and radish seeds, may be added for special flavoring and tastefulness.

A dressing over the salad of sprouts could be either sour cream, yogurt or a combination of sour cream, yogurt and cottage cheese. For an oil and vinegar dressing, add about one-quarter cup of good cider vinegar to a cup of sesame, sunflower or safflower oil. Walnut or peanut oil is also good and be sure to add a pinch of your favorite spice or herb, shaking the oil and vinegar together.

Dandelion leaves, chopped fine, may be sprinkled over the salad for additional taste and nourishment. Beet greens or mint leaves, such as spearmint, peppermint or catnip, may also be used. The leaves of young radish plants, cut or chopped, are also tasteful and nourishing.

For a healthful nonfattening drink to go with or follow the sprout salad, Beatrice mixes a cup of sprouts in the blender with two cups of pineapple juice. A half of banana with a slice of lemon is added for additional flavoring.

Other healthful, tasty and nonfattening drinks made by Beatrice include cutting up some wheat grass, about a cupful to one-half cup of water and placing the grass and the water in a blender for about a minute. The liquid is then strained and makes a healthful drink. The blender is also used to mix various fruits such as peaches, cantaloupe, apricots, strawberries and watermelon with orange juice, pineapple juice and a slice of lemon. There are unlimited other combinations.

THE TUESDAY AND FRIDAY SPROUTARIAN

I call John F. my Tuesday and Friday sproutarian. We had a consultation about his weight problem but he didn't want to go on a diet.

"What do you mean, you don't want to go on a diet?" I asked. "How do you expect to reduce if you don't go on a diet?"

John was 42 years old, weighed 220 pounds and was six feet tall. He was at least 40 pounds overweight.

"I enjoy food too much," he replied. "I don't want to go on a diet. But I'll make a deal with you. I'm willing to diet two days a week, provided you let me eat whatever I want to eat on the other five days of the week."

"It won't do any good," I countered, "unless you cut out the fatty foods."

"What fatty foods?" he asked, cautiously.

"First of all," I answered, "no dairy products such as milk, butter or cheese, but two eggs a day for breakfast are OK. However, no bacon, sausage or ham with your eggs. If you must have bread, it's got to be whole wheat."

"No butter on the bread?" he questioned.

"No butter."

"What about margarine?" he asked.

"Margarine, by law, must contain at least 80 percent fat. Also, many margarines have animal fat added to them and of course there is always yellow color added. If you must have something on your bread, which should be toasted for easier digestion, try a little yogurt or honey or a mixture of the two of them."

"What other restrictions will I need to observe during the five days of the week and what do I have to eat during the two days a week when I have to diet?"

"Avoid all fried foods, because fat is used in frying and the fat gets into the food. Avoid all food with sugar such as soft drinks, candy, sodas, pastries, ice cream, pies, chewing gum, cookies, cakes, donuts and a host of other products with sugar. Sugar can cause fatigue, hunger, obesity, migraine headaches, epilepsy, polio, alcoholism, asthma, heart trouble, constipation, skin diseases, teeth decay and many other problems. You can eat all you want except fatty foods, fried foods and foods containing sugar. As for dieting two days a week, that's easy. Just eat nothing but sprouts. Become a sproutarian! It's not too much to ask of you. Rather, you will be doing your body a favor. Sprouts contain practically all of the vitamins, minerals, protein and other nutritional elements that the body needs."

Believe it or not, within six weeks after our counseling session, John had lost those 40 pounds and was feeling fine. He was a Tuesday and Friday sproutarian.

COMBINING SPROUTS WITH OTHER FOODS

For a bright red salad, take a cup of alfalfa sprouts and mix with a cup of chopped red cabbage, a diced tomato, one large grated carrot, a cup of red onion slivers and about one-quarter cup of diced red pepper.

Prepare a cole slaw salad by mixing together one-half of a head of shredded cabbage with a half cup of green pepper, cut into small sections, one small onion and two cups of alfalfa sprouts.

School children will enjoy a peanut butter sandwich on whole wheat bread with an ample portion of alfalfa sprouts over the peanut butter and with some diced onions mixed in with the sprouts. It makes a fine snack for adults too.

For a healthy and sweet dessert with a minimum of fat-producing qualities, take almost any kind of sprout and grind or chop with almonds, cashews or other nuts and raisins, roll into small balls and then roll the balls over some shredded coconut.

Few people know that a potato, when thinly sliced, is quite palatable. A good combination is to mix some alfalfa sprouts with a thinly sliced potato, a cup of raw, sliced mushrooms and one-half cup of fresh peas.

A popular way of consuming sprouts is to drink them. Place a quantity of alfalfa sprouts into the blender with some chopped celery and chopped tomato, green pepper, cucumber and green onion. To liquefy, it will be necessary to add a liquid such as tomato juice, then blend it all together. If you want to avoid anything canned, place one or two fresh tomatoes into the blender at the start to obtain a liquid and then add the other ingredients one at a time.

For a sweet drink that will please kids and adults, cut up a pineapple and gradually liquefy it piece by piece in the blender. Add a cup of alfalfa sprouts and about a tablespoonful of honey and you have a delightfully sweet and nourishing drink.

If you have mint growing in your garden, throw in about ten mint leaves during the blending process and you will have a refreshing mint-flavored drink with a delightful fragrance as well.

The use of sprouting herb seeds results in the optimum value of the herb being absorbed into the human digestive system. The combinations for the use of sprouts with other healthful foods are innumerable. Mixing sprouts with low-fat cottage cheese is one way of obtaining excellent nourishment without adding body fat, thereby forcing the body to obtain fat from the body fat reserve. Yogurt is also an excellent food that may be added to sprout mixtures.

While there are many combinations involving heating in fry pans or bringing to a boil in a pot, it must be remembered that in order to fry it is necessary to add fat to the food to prevent burning and the fat is absorbed by the food and enters the digestive system. So far as boiling is concerned, water must reach a temperature of $212°$ F in order to boil and the live enzymes in food will be killed at about $140°$F. Eating food without enzymes forces the body to work hard to produce enzymes and this in turn causes an overworking and eventual nonfunctioning of the pancreas, where insulin is secreted.

The more simple and natural the food, the better it is for you.

Chapter Eleven

Using Herbal Spices for
Delicious Meals

The physician of the future will be he who keeps us from getting sick.
Thomas Alva Edison

THE greatest motivating factor for the use of herbs, aside from the tastefulness and fragrance added to food, is the fact that herbal spices help to keep the body well and prevent sickness. After all, it must be acknowledged that the medicines of today are largely derived from the herbs and spices in common use for medicinal purposes many years ago. You probably eat herbs daily, whether you know it or not, because a herb is any plant grown from seed that does not develop woody tissue. This definition includes many common vegetables which we have been eating for years without realizing the presence of important nutritional qualities.

UNUSUAL WAYS TO INCLUDE
AROMATIC HERBS IN YOUR DIET

Aromatic herbs are great for the skin and, through the skin, are absorbed into the bloodstream to some degree and provide nourishment and nutrition. In a sense, they become part of the diet.

In the ancient bathhouses, the rich Romans vied with each other in the use of the most valuable bath oils, at great expense. It is now within the reach of everyone to bathe in some of the fragrant aromatic herbs and spices such as jasmine, mint, lavender, lemon flowers, pennyroyal, lovage, camomile and elder leaves, berries, bark and flowers.

Of the aromatic herbs, jasmine has been popular for thousands of years, from the time of the ancient Hindus, when they were used to make neck garlands to show friendship. In Italy, it may still be the custom to entwine jasmine flowers into the bridal headdress, having been brought to Europe from the Far East sometime about the middle of the sixteenth century. The flowers make a healthful tea, and are said to be nourishing to muscle tissue and the nerves, relieving spasms and nerve pains.

There are many varieties of mint but they all share in the unique mint fragrance that makes bathing and tea drinking so pleasant. Not only does mint have cleansing and invigorating properties but the mint tea is commonly used as a digestive aid.

Pennyroyal is a form of mint, also used both in the bath and as a tea. Inhaling it during a cold is reported to be the most effective way of getting rid of a heavy cold.

Used as an herbal bath from earliest times, camomile has a fragrance that still makes it attractive both as a bath addition and as a fragrant and healthful tea. The old herbal books tell of the many virtues of camomile, allegedly helping various pains, strains and sprains and relieving toothaches as well as gas pains of the intestines.

The dried leaves and flowers of lavender, another variety of mint, are also valuable for bathing and for tea-making. As with other herbs and spices, do not throw the leaves or flowers into the bath water as you will have a hard time removing them from the body when you finish with your bath. Wrap the herbs, either singly or mixed with other herbs for a variety of fragrances, into a cheesecloth and allow it to soak in the tub. A smaller quantity, in a smaller piece of cheesecloth, may be used for soaking into the teacup.

Another aromatic bath, which is also of a nourishing nature and said to keep the body skin unwrinkled and youthful looking, is the herb known as houseleek, said to be used by the famous French beauty Ninon de Lenclos in combination with mint, lavender, thyme and rosemary. Houseleek is a pink-flowered plant found mainly on European old house rooftops and walls.

While lovage is not a highly aromatic herb, it is recognized as a deodorant and its use makes it feasible to avoid so many of the deodorants now on the market that contain a form of aluminum, said to have toxic effects on the body. Incidentally, aluminum cooking utensils should be avoided because it is said that aluminum contaminates the food.

Elder leaves, berries, bark and flowers, previously mentioned, have the effect, according to the old herbals, of soothing the nerves, helping to fall asleep, healing the eyes as well as sores of all kinds and bleaching and stimulating the skin.

Some other herbs that have an aroma are cinnamon, cloves, pepper, nutmeg, allspice and mace.

Use allspice in soups, cinnamon over fruits, cloves and pepper over eggs, potatoes, tomatoes, fish and over meat, mace over vegetables and nutmeg over chicken and vegetables.

These aromatic herbs are not only healthful but add a fragrance and aroma to food that makes eating the pleasure that it should be.

ADDING SWEETNESS TO FOODS WITH HERBS

In weaning yourself from the sickening and fattening habits of junk foods, so-called because although perhaps tasteful, they are worthless and have little or no nutritional value, it is important to seek ways and means of substituting tasty and sweet-tasting foods for the sweetness of sugary and fatty foods.

Perhaps most famous for its ability to sweeten food is fenugreek, originally from the Middle East, India and Southern Europe, and now cultivated in many other places. A teaspoonful of fenugreek seeds, dropped into a bowl of soup or spread over meat, fish, vegetables or other foods, will add a sweet taste that will fully satisfy your sweet tooth. It has recently been used as the principal flavoring of imitation maple syrup. The seeds may also be used as a tea. One old herbal claims that the tea is useful as a gargle for throat irritations.

Another help for overweights seeking to avoid the sweetness of fats and sugar products is to grow accustomed to the use of licorice. The common name of this herb is sweetwood; it was originally found in Southern Europe and Western Asia. The dried root is said to be four times sweeter than cane sugar. A teaspoonful of the powdered root into a cup of hot water makes a delicious tea. In addition to providing a sweet drink, there are especially beneficial side effects to overweight individuals as licorice reduces thirst and thereby prevents excessive drinking of fluids. Sugary products, on the other hand, increase thirst. Another beneficial side effect of licorice is its laxative effect and, additionally, the reported ability of this herb to eliminate or greatly reduce ulcers of the stomach and intestinal tract. It is also said to relieve coughs and sore throats.

Sweet marjoram is another excellent seasoning that imparts a sweet taste for satisfying the so-called sweet tooth. Not only does marjoram help digestion but it has been recommended for asthma and coughs. The leaves of the herb have an agreeable taste and have long been a favorite in kitchens as a seasoning.

Another herb, often referred to as sweet fennel, was cultivated by the ancient Romans and is found not only along the shores of the Mediterranean and in India but is also common in California. Not only does it have a pleasant taste but it is said to be especially effective in breaking down fatty tissue as well as conditions of accumulation of fluids in tissue. The leaves, seeds and root are all useful. The stems may be peeled and used as a salad, often served with a dressing of vinegar and pepper. The leaves, seeds or root may be boiled and made into a tea with a distinctive aroma and a sweetish milk and spicy taste. It is widely reported that drinking fennel tea helps to strengthen the eyesight.

While on the subject of eyesight, the use of sage tea has also been highly recommended for clearing the vision and strengthening the eyesight. In addition, it is also reported as benefiting the brain, nerves and glands. It is also said to greatly improve the memory. For a sweetening effect, add some honey. While sugar is not a food and is lacking in vitamins or minerals, honey contains iron, copper, manganese, silica, chlorine, calcium, potassium, sodium, phosphorus, aluminum and magnesium, all derived from the soil in which plants grow and, through the plant to the nectar, which is made into honey. Add some parsley to the sage drink for a mellowness to modify the spiciness of sage.

Shredded mint leaves may be added to practically any food or drink. While the flavor may not be "sweet" in the true sense of the word, the flavor is so appealing and the fragrance so pleasant that it is said to be the darling of the kitchen. It has long been used as a masking flavor, removing undesirable tastes from foods and drinks. Peppermint tea is widely used as a nightcap, being helpful to the digestion as well as helping to ward off or even relieve colds. Once the mint plants reach the flowering stage, the leaves become somewhat tough and the fragrance is greatly diminished. The young shoots should be cut after reaching two or three inches in height, for maximum aroma and taste.

The leaves of the herb known as sweet cicely, also known as sweet fern and as British myrrh, have a sugary essence that also classifies this plant as of the sweetness variety. It is an ancient plant, well known in Europe and believed to be a British native. The fruit, leaves and root are all used. The brownish-black fruits are flavorful and the root may be tenderized in boiling water and used as a vegetable. Even the seeds of this plant are used as a flavoring. Apparently, the plant heals the mucous membrane as it is recommended for healing coughs and pleurisy.

For thousands of years, violets and leaves of the violet plant have been enjoyed, long recognized as having a pleasant fragrance and a sweet taste. The violet flowers are boiled, cut or macerated, mixed with some warm milk and some honey added. This drink is said to be endowed with health-giving properties. To avoid the fattening effect of milk, use plain water instead and make a hot drink out of violet flowers, lemon and honey. It is said to be good for inducing a good sleep and helpful for cardiac conditions and ulcers. The leaves may also be added to the tea, after being cut into small pieces or shredded. Violets are propogated by seed, the use of runners and the employment of cuttings.

USING POWDERED HERBS IN SOUPS

In the powdering of herbs, bear in mind that the more processing of a food, the more the food loses its original qualities. It is generally accepted, for example, that fruits, vegetables or plants generally that have been cut, sliced, chopped or ground in any manner start to lose nutritional factors such as vitamins more quickly than if left whole. Minerals are not destroyed by the larger exposure to oxygen when a food is cut or chopped. In the case of iron, however, it is generally known that exposure to oxygen will cause erosion. The attraction of oxygen to iron while the plant is still whole results in a chemical action that allows the oxygen to be absorbed into the plant. The oxygen reaches the plant leaves and by combining with other compounds or elements creates chlorophyll.

The kind of powdered herb to use depends upon the nature of the soup you have on hand. Some soups are made entirely of vegetables, either mixed vegetables or only one vegetable. Other soups are made of poultry, meat or even a combination of poultry, meat and vegetables.

For vegetables soups, the most popular spices are allspice, anise seeds, celery seeds, chervil, cumin seeds, dill, garden burnet, oregano and rosemary.

For soups made with fish, use asafetida, chervil and garden marjoram.

For soups with meat, use asafetida, bay leaves, cumin seeds, garden marjoram and tarragon.

The fragrance and flavor of basil is such that it may be used with all varieties of soup.

For anyone wanting to reduce, beware of soup recipes that call for cream. Although the soup may acquire a rich taste by the addition of cream, substitute water for the cream. Also, ignore recipe instructions for adding sugar.

As a rule, soups are so full of vitamins and minerals that a good soup dish is a meal in itself. It is always better to undereat than to overeat, especially when you are careful enough to obtain your share of vitamins, minerals, protein and enzymes daily.

The use of salt has been purposely omitted, since an excessive salt content in the body tissue can bring about high blood pressure and death from brain hemorrhage. Besides, many foods contain salt in varying amounts. Animal foods usually have more salt than vegetables. Sea fish are higher in salt content than freshwater fish. Frozen fish, unless labeled as salt-free, are all high in salt. Also certain vegetables are salty, such as artichokes, beets, carrots, celery, chard, kale, spinach, dandelion greens, endive and corn.

However, the body does need a fair amount of salt and a completely salt-free diet may induce weakness, muscle cramps, low blood pressure and fatigue.

THE BOUQUET CONNECTION

You can make a bouquet of herbs, sometimes referred to as bouquets garnis. Take a mixture of dried herbs such as thyme, rosemary, sage, savory and marjoram for meat and vegetable soups. Use dill, basil, oregano, lemon balm, thyme and savory for fish stews and soups. Place the herbs into a cheesecloth sack and leave in the stew while cooking.

The proportions for the meat and vegetable food would be one part of thyme and sage to two parts of the other herbs mentioned. As for the fish dishes, the dill, oregano and thyme would be about one-half the quantity of the other herbs used.

HERBAL SPICES IN PLACE OF BUTTER

Learning how to make your own butter out of herbs and spices and other natural foods, instead of using fattening butter made from cream or using vegetable fats, is in itself a sufficient reason for the purchase of this book.

One delicious spread for bread is to take some prunes, put them in a small pan and cover with water. Bring the water to a boil, reduce the heat until you see the water just barely simmering. Leave the prunes in the pan until they are soft and tender. Shut off the heat and let the water cool for about 10 or 15 minutes. Remove the pits and save the juice in the refrigerator as a nourishing drink that will keep your bowels functioning regularly. Crush the remaining prunes with a potato masher or by mashing them on a board. If you have a blender, add a little apple cider vinegar and blend the prunes with the vinegar. Add a little nutmeg, allspice or powdered cloves to taste. You may want to use only one of these spices or all of them. You may also want to add a little honey for sweetening.

I usually avoid specifying exact quantities because people vary in their tastes. If you like one food or herb more than another, it is all right to use a little more of it. In making prune butter, it makes little difference as to the quantity because after you have mixed everything together, you will then put the mixture back in the pan for cooking until it is thick. It is then ready to smear over some homemade toasted whole wheat bread or any other good bread you may have on hand. Store the prune butter in the refrigerator and use as needed.

If you would rather have peach butter or if peaches are in season and available at low cost, use one portion of water to three portions of crushed peaches.

Prepare the peaches by first scalding them in boiling hot water for one minute. The skins will then be easily removable. After removing the skins and the pits, place the peaches in a pot and cook until they are soft on a low fire. Stir occasionally so the peaches do not stick to the bottom of the pot.

After the peaches are soft, mash them with a potato masher or in a blender and then add some grated nutmeg, powdered allspice or both, to suit your taste. Place in an oven at 325°F for one hour in an uncovered shallow roasting pan, stirring every 15 minutes until the butter is thick. Then pour into a jar and keep in the refrigerator for use as needed.

If you want to make lots of peach butter (or apricot butter) for storage purposes, ladle the butter into hot, sterilized jars. You can sterilize the jars by placing them in large pots of water and boiling the water for about ten minutes. Leave about one-quarter inch of space at the top of the jar before sealing and closing it. Finally, to kill any remaining bacteria, boil the sealed jars in the large pot for another ten minutes. After the jars cool, store in a cool, dry and dark place.

You can make plum butter too, for a change. You may even want to have two or three butters on hand and give each family member the choice of butter he or she wants to eat. Use the same procedure in making plum butter as in making prune or peach butter. Whether plums or other fruit, always remove any blemishes as well as pits and skins.

If grapes are plentiful, you may want to make some grape butter. Put the grapes in a pot with enough water to cover the grapes. While the water is simmering, mash the grapes. After the mixture thickens, you will want to remove the skins and the seeds and then continue the cooking until the mixture reaches the thickness of butter. Add some honey for sweetening. Spices may be added to all fruit butters for both aroma and taste.

An old favorite, apple butter, is just as easy to make as the other butters. Some recipes call for using apple cider instead of water. Remove the skin and core, stir frequently and simmer until the apple butter is a thick, dark brown mass. Cinnamon, allspice and ground cloves are the best spices to use.

While honey has been mentioned several times as a sweetener, it is best to first taste the butter before adding the honey, as it may already be sweet enough.

Pear butter can be made the same way as apple butter.

Chapter Twelve

How Juices Help
You Lose Weight

*Almost everyone is able to take raw fruits and vegetables in liquid form,
and these liquefied salads are also easy to make.*

Dr. Bernard Jensen

THE popularity of the blender has made the liquefying of food easier for digestion. Chewing breaks the food down so it is more easily assimilated into the body. It should be sipped rather than swallowed, so as to allow the salivary juices to mix with the liquid.

This chapter continues to emphasize the importance of achieving daily an intake of all the needed nutritional elements of the body. The blender does a superb job of masticating food, better than teeth. However, the mastication of food breaks open and exposes to the air the tiny food particles intended to nourish various parts of the body. Unless entering the digestive system without delay, there is a tendency for the exposure to the air to cause a deterioration in food value.

HOW TO DRINK LIQUIDS FOR WEIGHT REDUCTION

Just as we are careful in selecting our solid foods to prevent adding fat to our bodies, so do we need to take care in preparing liquid drinks to select foods that will take weight off.

The same vitamins, minerals, proteins, fats and carbohydrates that exist in solid foods also exist in liquids. The information and knowledge we have gained with respect to the values of solid foods applies with equal strength to foods that have been liquefied.

Of course, the size of an orange as compared with the size of orange juice made from that same orange has a substantial difference. It would be easy to drink in excess, just as it is easy to eat solid food in excess. For anyone interested in weight reduction, therefore, keep in mind that juice quantities are rich and concentrated with the food values.

Timing is also important. If you are accustomed to spending an hour at the dining table, do not plan to spend the same amount of time partaking of juices. Even with slow sipping, the time drinking juices would probably be only one-fourth of the time spent eating solid foods.

On a recent motor-home trip, I prepared a salad of vegetables and made enough for three days. My entire luncheons for those three days consisted of one cup of the liquefied salad.

You may be interested to know what the salad ingredients were. They included romaine lettuce, spinach, asparagus, carrots, alfalfa sprouts, a tomato, brussel sprouts, celery, parsley and one green onion. While some of the good food values deteriorated somewhat waiting in the refrigerator, the deterioration was not so substantial as to require the making of fresh drinks daily.

I should mention that in my own case I am not overweight, weighing a slim 168 pounds with a height of six feet and one inch. According to the weight tables, I am just slightly underweight, which is the way I want to keep it.

One of the great advantages of liquid dieting is that spices and herbs may be freely intermingled to produce flavor and taste that is delightful. Needless to say, the health benefits make life more beautiful than ever before.

THE SUPERIORITY OF JUICES
OVER THE RAW PRODUCT

There is no tastier drink than a delicious fruit cocktail. In too many homes, it is the custom for the man of the house to stop at a tavern on his way home for a cold beer. If he knew that a freshly made fruit drink would be awaiting his arrival at home, the tavern stop would be more apt to be eliminated. If the weather is hot, add an ice cube to the blender mixture. Use some herbal spices to add a special tang to the drink. For fruits, use some allspice, which has a taste similar to a combination of cloves, cinnamon and nutmeg.

Then there is the matter of economy. Many vegetables come in packages and, with a small family, the package may be too large for a raw food salad, especially when a variety is desired. By cutting the vegetable into small pieces and making juice, waste can be more easily avoided. Even under refrigeration, food will spoil. It is best to go shopping frequently and get the food fresh rather than buy in large quantities and allow the food to deteriorate. Often, a market will lower the price on fruits and vegetables that are fully ripe and are about to spoil. These foods are at the peak of nutritive and taste value and if juiced without delay there is the double advantage of good health and economy.

Another advantage of juicing is the time factor. It takes time to set up a pretty salad dish, arranged just right with colors in balance and a rational pattern of placement of foods. It also takes time to wield that knife and fork to slice the vegetables into just the right sizes for lifting into the mouth. And it takes time to chew and chew and chew to break up the food particles into a more or less juicy substance so that it can be swallowed without choking and easily digested. On the other hand, a few seconds in a blender, with just a little water added to get the blender working, produces a liquid salad that can be swallowed much more quickly than the solid food. Of course, sipping a little at a time is preferable, so as to allow the salivary juices to mix with the food.

HOW HARRY K. LOST FOUR POUNDS A WEEK WITH CRANBERRY JUICE

Harry was quite overweight then I first met him. He was about five feet, seven inches tall and 38 years old. His weight should have been not more than 147 pounds but he weighed 180 pounds.

He ate and drank everything, especially beer. When I suggested to him that he stop eating junk foods and get on to a health program, he said that he liked fruit juices.

I suggested cranberry juice to him because it contains vitamin A, several good B vitamins (thiamine, riboflavin and niacin), vitamin C, and also some protein, fat, carbohydrates, calcium, iron and phosphorus. I also urged him to use pure, unprocessed, uncooked honey for sweetening as there are a wide range of nutrients in honey and some nutritionists believe it to be a complete food.

Relying upon what I had told him, Harry decided to go on a cranberry juice fast for one week. Here is how he prepared his juice: For each serving, he would take two-thirds of a cup of raw cranberries, rinse them and place them in a blender. He would then add two tablespoons of pure, unprocessed honey and the juice of one-half lemon. Lemons and other citrus fruits produce an alkaline reaction in the body, which will offset to some degree the acidity of the cranberries. One-half cup of distilled or filtered water was then added to the blender so that the blades would have something to beat when the current was turned on.

After liquefying the berries, Harry would sip the drink slowly and enjoy. He would take this drink several times a day to quench both hunger and thirst.

Harry found that he was not only able to lose an average of a pound a day over a week's time but he was able to maintain his strength and energy and in fact felt better than ever before.

There are some writers who have attributed marvelous healing benefits to cranberries but the health benefits of cranberries as well as other foods and plants will be the subject of a separate book some day. Researchers believe that cranberries help high blood pressure conditions, obesity, constipation, skin diseases, fever, kidney and liver problems, sore throats, diabetes and many other illnesses.

After the experimental week was over, Harry found that his weight was down to 173 pounds and he felt fine. He wanted to continue with the program and I agreed. However, I advised him to have some oatmeal in the morning after taking his cranberry juice and obtain some raw milk, preferably nonfat, to pour over it. This would add greatly to the necessary vitamins, protein, carbohydrates and minerals the body needs each day. I suggested he try sprinkling his cereal with some pumpkin pie seasoning, which is a blend of ground cinnamon, cloves, ginger and nutmeg.

There were times, he told me, that he would get especially hungry. When this happened he would make a little bowl of oatmeal and this would remove any craving for food.

As the days and weeks went on, I allowed him to get onto a more normal diet such as allowing a soft-boiled egg daily for breakfast and some alfalfa sprouts for lunch or snacking whenever there was any desire for food.

The results were simply marvelous. Weight reduction was rapid and without any ill effects. Harry took long walks early in the morning and sometimes in the evening twilight and was able to keep his muscles in good shape. He lost weight regularly and in just a little over a month was down to a weight of 145 pounds.

Incidentally, I also advised Harry to sprinkle some capsicum (commonly known as African bird pepper) liberally upon the soft-boiled egg. The rich vitamin C content of this red pepper helped him to ward off colds. In addition, his heart was stimulated to more activity, improving circulation throughout the body. This action on the body is also said to improve fertility and delay senility. There is a high potassium content in red pepper and this is very helpful to persons having edema or swelling of tissue. Many overweight persons have this problem.

THE SLIMMING QUALITIES OF VEGETABLE JUICES

When I speak of vegetable juices, I am referring to freshly made juices from ripe vegetables and not the canned variety. I have previously pointed out in my book, *Encyclopedia of Fruits, Vegetables, Nuts and Seeds for Healthful Living,* that the body needs the enzymes from live food.

Canning food requires that vegetables having a low-acid content must be heated for a longer time than high-acid foods such as apples, peaches and other fruits. The canning factories place the vegetables into steam pressure cookers that raise the temperature of the vegetables until it is hotter than boiling water

For example, in the sterilization of cream-style corn, it takes 160 minutes of cooking at a temperature of 240°F to kill all the organisms in the food.

The use of frozen vegetables for juicing is much better than the use of canned vegetables. Freezing does not sterilize the food but the extreme cold does stop the growth of organisms and the enzyme activity is greatly slowed down. The color, flavor and texture of vegetables or other foods that are frozen are preserved better than in the canning process.

What about using dried vegetables? Drying food is one of the oldest methods of preserving foods. Many years before Columbus discovered America, American Indians would dry fruits, vegetables, fish and meat. After drying, the meat would be pounded into a powder and used when fresh meat was not available.

Without water, bacteria and molds that usually form on unprocessed food cannot multiply or grow and so dried food will not spoil. Foods are dried by the sun or by dehydration. Commercial dehydration is done by placing the food on trays in compartments with moderate heat and low humidity. Air currents are machine-produced to assist in the dehydration. Many small and inexpensive drying cabinets are available and may be used to dry various foods.

To make vegetable juices, therefore, avoid the canned vegetables, but you may use the frozen vegetables or add water to the dried vegetables and then juice them. When adding water, try to avoid tap water and instead use bottled water, distilled water or water that has been filtered.

Tap water usually has had chemicals added to it to destroy organisms. Those same chemicals, when taken into the body, will destroy the organisms needed by the body for normal food absorption and digestion. The drinking of water loaded with destructive chemicals may be compared to breathing in a smoke-filled room. It is really dangerous to the body.

My fruit and vegetable book, mentioned previously, tells of the nutritive values of various fruits, vegetables, nuts and seeds, and this book would be too bulky were it to include all of the beneficial values of the various vegetables. It should be sufficient to say that vegetables contain all the vitamins and minerals and are therefore an easy and delightful way to meet all of the body needs and keep away from fattening foods.

Vegetable drinks are made, of course, in a blender, which is an indispensable aid for every kitchen. You will be surprised how solid vegetables such as carrots, asparagus, broccoli, lettuce, parsley and cauliflower are easily ground into a liquid form without any waste.

While the vegetables themselves have a unique taste and fragrance that makes them easy to swallow, this is a fine way to add herbs and spices into the vegetable juices. Some of the more popular herbs and spices are chili powder, curry powder, cardomom and Italian seasoning. Also, experiment with other spices such as ginger, basil, dill weed and rosemary.

Finally, you will need some liquid at the bottom of the blender to get started. I like to put in a tomato or two in the blender by itself to produce a liquid. Then, when the solid vegetables are added, a little at a time, the liquefying continues without any problems. Sometimes, I will use a little grape juice for the required liquid base. As a last resort, I will use some good water.

WHAT PAULA W. CALLED HER TOMATO-JUICE DIET

Paula W. was truly the five-by-five type when she started her tomato-juice diet. She was only five feet tall and seemed to be about five feet in diameter, weighing 175 pounds when, at the most, she should have weighed 115 pounds. Her so-called tomato-juice diet enabled her to reduce from 3 to 5 pounds a week and she lost all of her 60 pounds of fat in a little over four months. She is now 51 years old.

The last time I saw her, she was playing tennis, swimming and feeling fine.

"Paula," I said to her. "You know I'm writing a new book on weight loss with the use of herbs and spices and I would like to mention your case in my book. Would you please tell me how you did it?"

"It was easy," she responded, laughingly. "I just followed the teachings in your book on fruits, vegetables, nuts and seeds."

"Now, wait a minute," I protested. "My fruit and vegetable book only told of the values of foods and very little was given about actual recipes. And you certainly cannot have a well-balanced diet simply by drinking tomato juice."

"Let me explain," she said. "I did not use the canned tomato juice at all. As you know canned foods have to be heated in the canning process and all bacteria are destroyed. Therefore, I use one large tomato or two small fresh tomatoes."

"I can see that tomatoes will give you a fair amount of vitamin A, about 1100 international units per serving, but everyone over the age of ten should get at least 4000 units daily," I pointed out.

"That's true," she replied. "But I have my juice several times a day, and in addition, I add a couple of carrots, cut up into pieces, into the blender. The carrots get converted into a juice and add about 12,000 international units of vitamin A to my drink."

Chapter Thirteen

Some Special Hints
for Losing Weight

If you give nature half a chance it will bless you in many ways.

Dr. Philip J. Welsh

TIME after time, it has been shown beyond doubt that it is nature that heals, not the doctors, the hospitals or the drugs. We need to concentrate more and more on the use of natural foods, especially those free from preservatives, without any sugar content, saturated fats, white flour products or artificial flavoring.

HERBS USED IN WEIGHT-LOSS CASES

There have been many reports of persons who have used various herbs in weight-loss programs, in combination with avoidance of fattening foods. One such herb is cleavers. It is known to be a diuretic, facilitating the movement of liquid from the bladder, a tonic and a bowel stimulant. Taken three times daily as a tea, usually between meals over a period of several weeks, should show results in weight loss without any side effects.

There is a report of a woman who reduced from 210 pounds to 140 pounds, after several months of using fennel seed tea. This patient entered into a diet that was low on starches, sugars and fats. Fennel seeds are known to be rich in vitamin A. The tea is prepared by placing a teaspoonful of the seeds into a cup and then pouring hot water over the seeds. It is then allowed to steep and is taken three or four times a day.

Some reducing experts praise kelp as a very effective means of reducing. The taste of kelp is not pleasing but it is available in capsule or tablet form and takes effect after it is swallowed. Two or three tablets a day should suffice.

A product derived mainly from soybeans has been highly recommended for the use of overweight persons. The product, lecithin, attacks fatty deposits which seem to melt away for the lecithin user. It comes in liquid form and is not unpleasant. Two or three teaspoonfuls a day ought to get good results.

Raspberry leaf tea is a somewhat of a newcomer among reducing drinks. Your nearby health-food store probably has a supply of this herb. Drink two or three cups of tea daily. I usually add some lemon juice and a little honey to the herb teas that I drink. The tea, itself, will not do the trick, however. It is still vitally important to avoid fatty foods and to obtain all of the daily nutrients needed.

A fruit drink that has been highly recommended for reducing is grape juice. The famous herbalist Edgar Cayce spoke often of grape juice for reducing, urging the use of four glasses of grape juice daily before meals and before retiring.

A FEW WORDS ABOUT SALT

Salt and salted foods such as potato chips, pretzels, peanuts and crackers, as well as salt-preserved foods such as ham, bacon and pickles, should be avoided. Salt increases the flow of saliva, thereby increasing the appetite. In addition, it tends to hold water in the body and aggravates the weight problem. The late Adelle Davis, famous nutritionist, advised the use of potassium chloride, sold as a salt substitute, for persons wishing to reduce.

I recommend the free use of zesty herbs and spices for flavoring of food as better than a salt substitute. Experiment with ginger, rosemary, oregano, tarragon, cloves, sage, allspice, caraway, dill and many others.

These herbs do not have the salt effect of adding unnecessary fluid to the body. Try sprinkling oregano, paprika or tarragon on eggs, basil on tomatoes, pepper, ground rosemary or ginger on roasts (before broiling), powdered mint or cayenne on veal, savory or chili powder on green beans and allspice on squash or potatoes. Use basil on tomatoes and also for flavoring meat loaf. Get little containers with various herbs and spices in them and place them on the table during meals.

High blood pressure, strokes (caused by blood clots in the brain or in blood vessels in the heart area) are virtually unknown where little salt is used. Some salt is desirable but the salt needed is usually obtained from the eating of ocean fish or kelp, the sea vegetation so richly endowed with many minerals and vitamins, including iodine.

THE PROBLEMS OF THE ELDERLY LUCY M.

Lucy M. had just reached retirement age and was starting to receive her Social Security checks. Her problem was that all her life she had been a slave to "custom." It was customary to drink milk, so she drank it often all of her lifetime and acquired a lot of fat. It was customary to spread heavy coatings of butter or margarine over her bread, with overlays of cream cheese and jelly, which didn't help her overweight problem.

In addition, she ate lots of breads, cookies and donuts and had bacon, sausage or ham with her eggs every morning, plus lunch meats for lunch and meat and potatoes or poultry for dinner. She little realized that excess carbohydrates (flour products and potatoes) as well as excess protein turn into fat. Eating bread and protein with all three meals was just too much for her.

At a little over five feet tall, an ideal weight for Lucy would be about 125 pounds. Unfortunately, she had acquired a weight of 180 pounds and just did not know how to get rid of that extra poundage. She adored fatty foods and the dishes her mother had prepared during her childhood years. As to the dangers of fat, Lucy was still being visited by her over-eighty mother, who had long-thrived on the diet on which Lucy was reared and was in such spry good health that Lucy had difficulty in believing that her diet was not good.

"How are you doing, Lucy?" I asked. "Are you winning the battle of the bulge?"

"I've been fighting off those temptations," she answered, "but it's hard."

"Have you been following my advice about using spices to add taste and flavor to your meals, thereby providing a substitute for the fattening foods you are so accustomed to eating?"

"You bet I have!" she replied. "Remember how I told you that I just couldn't break away from the cheesecake habit? I used to make cheesecake with the richest cream cheese that I am sure added two or three pounds to my weight every time I made one. Well, I found a substitute cake that is even more delicious, made with healthful spices, and without any fattening ingredients. Want to know the recipe?"

She told me how to do it. She used whole wheat pastry flour and sour cream with two eggs, nutmeg, cloves and cinnamon to make a cake that not only satisfied her sweet tooth but convinced her that it is possible to enjoy delicious cake without putting on weight.

First, she would preheat the oven to 350° F and spread some safflower oil over an 8 × 8-inch square pan. She would then beat two egg yolks, add about one-third cup of honey, a cup of sour cream and mix these ingredients well. She would then combine one and one-half cups of whole wheat pastry flour with a teaspoon of baking soda, one-quarter teaspoon of kosher salt, one-quarter teaspoon of nutmeg, one-quarter teaspoon of ground cloves and one-half teaspoon of cinnamon. This mixture would then be combined with the first mixture of the wet ingredients. Some raisins may be added for additional taste and flavor. Two egg whites, stiffly beaten, should then be added.

Pour it all into the pan and bake for 35 or 45 minutes. Make sure the cake is ready by piercing it with a knife after 35 minutes. If the knife is dry, the cake is ready.

I congratulated Lucy on using this cake in substitution for cheesecake and asked her if she had learned some other ways of changing over to nonfattening meals.

"You won't believe this," she half-whispered with enthusiasm, "but I now bake my own breadsticks and I've learned how to cover them with sesame, poppy and caraway seeds. My family just loves them!"

"Do you use whole wheat flour?"

"Not only do I use whole wheat flour but I've bought a grinder and I buy the wheat berries and grind them as I need flour," she responded, to my great surprise.

Wheat berry grinders do not come cheap and it is hard to get people to realize that by having your own grinder you can make all kinds of breads, rolls and cakes at considerable savings when compared with the high store prices. In the long run, having your own grinder saves money. You can also grind corn, rice, soybeans and other seeds.

For use in baking bread, the ordinary grind of red winter wheat is fine but use whole wheat pastry flour if you want to bake biscuits, breadsticks or cake. For this type of flour, you will want to use the soft wheat instead of the hard wheat. Grind the wheat berries as finely as you can and then grind it a second time to make it extra fine. It should be sifted to lighten the flour and let air get into it.

Bran from the flour will drop to the bottom of the sifter but should be returned to the sifted flour so that the whole wheat flour will retain all of its value. The natural whole flour contains about 20 different substances, some of which have not yet been isolated and identified. However, scientists believe that the healthiest food is the natural food. The wheat germ in wheat is of especially high value. However, wheat germ is perishable, and it is best to keep whole wheat ground flour in the refrigerator to prevent spoilage.

"Just how do you prepare these spicy breadsticks?" I asked.

"It's easy," Lucy replied. "You will need a package of dry yeast. Dissolve the yeast in some lukewarm water, using about one-half cup of water for this purpose. Then pour about one-half cup of safflower oil into a large bowl with one and one-half tablespoons of honey. Add a teaspoon of kosher salt (said to be most natural and unrefined) to the bowl with one-half cup of boiling water. After this mixture has cooled somewhat, add one beaten egg and then the dissolved yeast. Gradually stir into the bowl about three and one-half cups of whole wheat pastry flour and mix well.

"When whole wheat flour is mixed with yeast, the dough does not have to be kneaded, which just suits me fine," said Lucy, smiling broadly. "After the ingredients are mixed, the dough is allowed to rise once in the pan. If the dough being made is too watery, more flour should be added to remove the watery feeling.

"In baking breadsticks, I have found it best to place the dough into the refrigerator for about 10 minutes, right after making the dough," she said. "While it is in the refrigerator, I will turn on the oven to 425° F so as to let it preheat. I will then take the dough out of refrigeration and divide it into 12 equal parts. I then roll the pieces of dough on a floured board, making each breadstick about one-half inch in diameter.

"I like to use safflower oil for all baking needs because of the absence of animal fats and preservatives. I will then spread some of this oil on a baking sheet. After placing the breadsticks on the pan, about one and one-half inches apart, I will sprinkle them with sesame seeds, poppy seeds or caraway seeds."

Lucy added that sometimes she would use all of the seeds, adding some variety of seed to some sticks and other breadsticks would be given other varieties of seeds.

"Just for fun and variety," Lucy added, "I will sprinkle some finely cut pieces of onion onto the breadsticks and I've also tried sticking raisins on them and small pieces of garlic. The kids just love to try out different flavors and, of course, I do too."

Incidentally, you may have noticed that in describing how to bake her cake with spices Lucy made no mention of yeast or baking powder. She had learned that the proportion of one teaspoon of baking soda to a cup of buttermilk or sour cream imparts a rising quality to the dough so as to make yeast or baking powder unnecessary.

The baking soda is alkaline and the buttermilk or sour cream is acid and it is in the combination of the two that the leavening or rising effect is produced. Should a recipe be used that does not have such a combination, baking powder may be homemade by mixing two teaspoons of cream of tartar with one teaspoon of bicarbonate of soda and adding one-half teaspoon of salt, for every cup of flour in the recipe. It is the heat from the hot oven that brings about most of the rising action.

Lucy spoke of adding raisins, onion and garlic to the breadsticks by sprinkling over the dough. I told her that these items could be added to the dough mixture as well and would be more likely to preserve their taste, fragrance and food value.

"What else have you been doing to reduce your weight?" I asked Lucy.

"I've learned how to make a whole meal out of a salad," she replied.

Lucy explained that after preparing a salad composed of lettuce, tomato slices, green pepper, celery or a variety of other vegetables she would add to it some pieces of cold chicken, turkey, beef tongue, or sliced hard-boiled eggs. Sometimes she would use radishes, chopped olives, sardines, grated carrots, grated or sliced onions, green onions and horseradish.

For a salad dressing, she would make her own version of a thousand island dressing. Into a cup of tomato juice, she would add two tablespoons of tarragon vinegar, a teaspoon of onion juice, a half-teaspoon of fresh basil, two teaspoons of chopped parsley, a few grains of cayenne, a clove of garlic chopped into small pieces and a chopped hard-boiled egg. There was nothing fattening and I agreed with her that the taste and fragrance was simply grand.

Lucy cut her weight in six months from 180 pounds to 140 pounds. Her target is 125 pounds and she should reach it soon. She avoids all fattening foods, products made with white flour or sugar, caffeine-containing foods or drinks, including the cola drinks and fried foods.

HOW VEGETARIAN CHARLES S. GETS HIS PROTEIN

Charles S. and I play tennis often. When I first met him, he was truly obese, weighing about 70 pounds more than he should. At age 55, he weighed 250 pounds whereas he should have weighed not more than 180 pounds at the most. He is five feet, 11 inches tall.

After several conversations, Charles decided to become a vegetarian. This was more than I had anticipated because I have never felt that vegetarianism is the answer. However, I did not discourage him because if the vegetarian can get enough protein, it is not really a bad regimen.

He lost 70 pounds at the rate of two pounds a week. He could have reduced more rapidly but was afraid of a sudden weight loss. Besides, he felt fine, enjoyed food and wanted to make the changeover gradually.

"I'm in no hurry to lose weight," he frequently said. "I'm feeling fine. I know that it's important to reduce and I'm going to do it but in my own good time."

No matter what I told him about the urgency to reduce rapidly—how he had no time to lose, how all that extra weight was a burden on his heart, how the diet he was on was slowly poisoning him—it would do no good unless he became convinced of the need for reducing as rapidly as possible, with due regard to his bodily needs for the day's activities.

I invited him to attend a series of free public lectures on health and nutrition I was giving at the local public library. He started attending and learning and the more he learned, the more weight he lost. Soon he became so interested that he started to concoct some original vegetable and herb combinations.

"People talk about the value of milk for the purpose of getting calcium," Charles would say. "They don't know that leafy green vegetables, soybeans, sunflower and sesame seeds are abundant sources of calcium. Alfalfa tea is also rich in calcium and provides a nourishing and tasty drink as well, especially if you add a little lemon and honey."

He is right! One glass of milk contains only 300 milligrams of calcium while three ounces of sesame seeds contain 1,125 milligrams. Only one ounce of these seeds would provide more calcium than a glass of milk. Think of all the fat you get with milk that you do not get with sesame seeds or alfalfa tea.

"Are you getting enough protein?" I asked. A sufficient amount of protein for vegetarians always worried me.

"Well, that's always a problem for a vegetarian," he grumbled. "I know that nuts contain lots of protein but as a rule they usually contain a lot of fat, too, so I eat them but only a small amount. I eat lots of barley, beans and chickpeas. Barley provides about 8 grams to a serving, beans about 7½ grams and chickpeas pay off with about 21 grams to a serving. Dulse is also rich in protein, with about 25 grams in a serving of about 100 grams. This food also contains iron, iodine, phosphorus, potassium and calcium."

"Are you familiar with the rule about the amount of protein that you need daily?" I asked.

"Sure," he replied quickly. "You just divide your weight by two and that tells you how many grams of protein you need daily. I weigh 180 pounds so I need 90 grams of protein daily."

"Do you get that many each day?"

"Probably not, but I try. I try to pick out foods that have lots of protein as well as other nutritive factors such as vitamins and minerals. Oats, millet and mature peas are all rich in protein and when I eat bread I generally choose rye or whole wheat bread. Rye and wheat are rich in protein too, besides containing several of the vitamins in the B complex and relatively large quantities of calcium, iron and phosphorus. Soybeans contain a lot of protein as do sesame seeds. The vitamin E in sesame seeds strengthens the heart and nervous system."

I was highly pleased with his enumeration of the protein-carrying foods. It was clear to me that he was a good student. I have often emphasized in my lectures the importance of locating and using foods rich in protein if you are going to be a vegetarian. Charles had learned his lessons well.

Index